INTERMEDIATE FETAL MONITORING COURSE

Student Materials

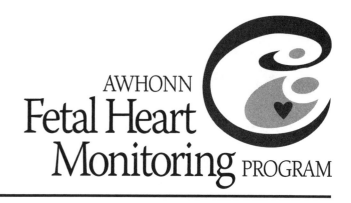

AWHONN
Fetal Heart
Monitoring PROGRAM

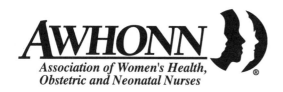

AWHONN
Association of Women's Health,
Obstetric and Neonatal Nurses

KENDALL/HUNT PUBLISHING COMPANY
4050 Westmark Drive   Dubuque, Iowa 52002

Cover image © JupiterImages Corporation, Inc.

Copyright © 1993, 1997, 2003, 2006 by Association of Women's Health, Obstetric and Neonatal Nurses

ISBN 978-0-7575-2807-1

Printed in the United States of America
10 9 8 7 6 5 4 3

CONTENTS

INTRODUCTION AND SUPPLEMENTAL INFORMATION

Target Audience

The Intermediate Fetal Monitoring Course is designed for healthcare professionals with a minimum of six months clinical experience using fetal heart monitoring technology in an intrapartum setting. It is expected that the participant already have basic knowledge and related skills in the following areas:

- Maternal physiologic changes of pregnancy.
- Fetal growth and development.
- Methods of fetal monitoring.
- Preparation of patient for setup and initiation of external or internal fetal monitoring.
- Obtaining and maintaining tracings that document fetal heart rate and uterine contractions.
- Interpretation of uterine contraction frequency, duration and baseline resting tone.
- Identification of the baseline fetal heart rate, variability, and deviations.
- Indicated clinical interventions.
- Communication and documentation standards.

Acknowledgement of Commercial Support

This CNE/CME activity has been created without commercial support.

Sponsorship Statement

This CNE activity is co-sponsored by the Association of Women's Health, Obstetric and Neonatal Nurses (AWHONN) and by the Professional Education Services Group (PESG).

Learning Objectives

At the conclusion of this continuing medical education activity, participants should be able to:

- Demonstrate the decision-making process necessary for the proper selection and verification of fetal heart monitoring (FHM) techniques.
- Analyze fetal heart rate patterns, uterine activity and their implications for fetal well-being.
- Correlate indicated clinical interventions with related maternal-fetal physiology.
- Describe the role and responsibility of the professional nurse in the use of FHM in intrapartum care.
- Simulate the psychomotor skills used in FHM.
- Communicate verbal and written data about patient status and verify accountability.

Content Validation Statement

It is the policy of AWHONN and PESG to review and certify that the content contained in this CNE/CME activity is based on sound, scientific, evidence-based medicine. All recommendations involving clinical medicine in this CNE/CME activity are based on evidence that is accepted within the profession of medicine as adequate justification for their indications and contraindications in the care of patients.

AWHONN and PESG further assert that all scientific research referred to, reported, or used in this CNE/CME activity in support or justification of a patient care recommendation conforms to the generally accepted standards of experimental design, data collection, and analysis. Moreover, AWHONN and PESG establishes that the content contained herein conforms to the Definition of CNE as defined by the American Nurses Credentialing Center (ANCC) and the Definition of CME as defined by the Accreditation Council for Continuing Medical Education (ACCME).

Disclosure Statement

It is the policy of Professional Education Services Group that the faculty and sponsor disclose real or apparent conflicts of interest relating to the topics of this educational activity and also disclose discussions of unlabeled/unapproved uses of drugs or devices during their presentations. Detailed disclosures will be made available during the live program.

Conflict-of-Interest Resolution Statement

When individuals in a position to control content have reported financial relationships with one or more commercial interests, as listed in their particular disclosure, AWHONN and PESG will work with them to resolve such conflicts to ensure that the content presented is free from commercial bias. The content of this presentation was vetted by the following mechanisms and modified as required to meet this standard:

- Content peer review by external topic expert
- Content validation by external topic expert and internal AWHONN and PESG clinical staff
  Educational Peer Review Disclosure PESG reports the following:

- **William Mencia, MD**,
  Vice President of Medical Affairs/CME Director
  Dr. Mencia has no significant financial relationships to disclose.

- **Lawrence Devoe, MD**
  Dr. Devoe has no significant financial relationships to disclose.

Accreditation Information

AWHONN is accredited as a provider of continuing nursing education (CNE) in nursing by the American Nurses Credentialing Center's Commission on Accreditation.

AWHONN also holds California and Alabama BRN numbers: California CE provider # CEO 580 and Alabama # ABNP0058.

The maximum CNE credit that can be earned while attending the Intermediate Fetal Monitoring Course is 18 AWHONN contact hours.

Professional Education Services Group is accredited by the Accreditation Council for Continuing Medical Education (ACCME) to provide continuing medical education for physicians. This activity has been planned and implemented in accordance with the Essential Areas and policies of the ACCME.

Credit Designation Statement

Physicians: Professional Education Services Group designates this educational activity for a maximum of 15.25 category 1 credits toward the AMA Physician's Recognition Award. Each physician should claim only those credits that he/she actually spent in the activity.

DISCLAIMER

This course and all accompanying materials (publication) were developed by AWHONN, the Association of Women's Health, Obstetric and Neonatal Nurses, as an educational resource for fetal heart monitoring. It presents general methods and techniques of practice that are currently acceptable, based on current research and used by recognized authorities. Proper care of individual patients may depend on many individual factors to be considered in clinical practice, as well as professional judgment in the techniques described herein. Clinical circumstances naturally vary, and professionals must use their own best judgment in accordance with the patients' needs and preferences, professional standards and institutional rules. Variations and innovations that are consistent with law, and that demonstrably improve the quality of patient care, should be encouraged.

AWHONN has sought to confirm the accuracy of the information presented herein and to describe generally accepted practices. However, neither AWHONN nor PESG are responsible for errors or omissions or for any consequences from application of the information in this resource and makes no warranty, expressed or implied, with respect to the contents of the publication.

Competent clinical practice depends on a broad array of personal characteristics, training, judgment, professional skills and institutional processes. This publication is simply one of many information resources. This publication is not intended to replace ongoing evaluation of knowledge and skills in the clinical setting. Nor has it been designed for use in hiring, promotion or termination decisions or in resolving legal disputes or issues of liability.

AWHONN and PESG believe that drug selection and dosage set forth in this text are in accordance with current recommendations and practice at the time of publication. However, in view of ongoing research, changes in government regulations, and the constant flow of information relating to drug therapy and drug reactions, the reader is urged to check other information available in other published sources for each drug for potential changes in indications, dosages, and for added warnings, and precautions. This is particularly important when the recommended agent is a new or infrequently employed drug. In addition, appropriate medication use may depend on unique factors such as individuals' health status, other medication use, and other factors which the professional must consider in clinical practice.

RESOURCES AND REFERENCE MATERIALS

BASELINE VARIABILITY

The numbers (1) through (4) included in the following cells correspond to the numbers encircled on the Visual Assessment of Variability Scale.

Amplitude of FHR Change	Former AWHONN Baseline LTV Description	NICHD Baseline Variability Description
(1) Undetectable from baseline	Decreased/Minimal	Absent
(2) Visually detectable from baseline, ≤5 bpm	Decreased/Minimal	Minimal
(3) 6–25 bpm	Average/Within Normal Limits	Moderate
(4) >25 bpm	Marked/Saltatory	Marked

Source: Adapted from Electronic fetal heart monitoring: Research guidelines for interpretation, National Institutes of Child Health and Human Development Research Planning Workshop, 1997, *Journal of Obstetric, Gynecologic and Neonatal Nursing, 26*(6), 635–640. Copyright © AWHONN.

Note: The exact language in the 1997 NICHD paper regarding minimal variability is "greater than undetectable" and less than or equal to 5 bpm. AWHONN has chosen the equivalent term "visually detectable" to clearly differentiate the definition of minimal variability from the definition of "absent variability," avoid confusion for users new to the NICHD terminology, and emphasize the visual determination of variability.

VISUAL ASSESSMENT OF VARIABILITY SCALE

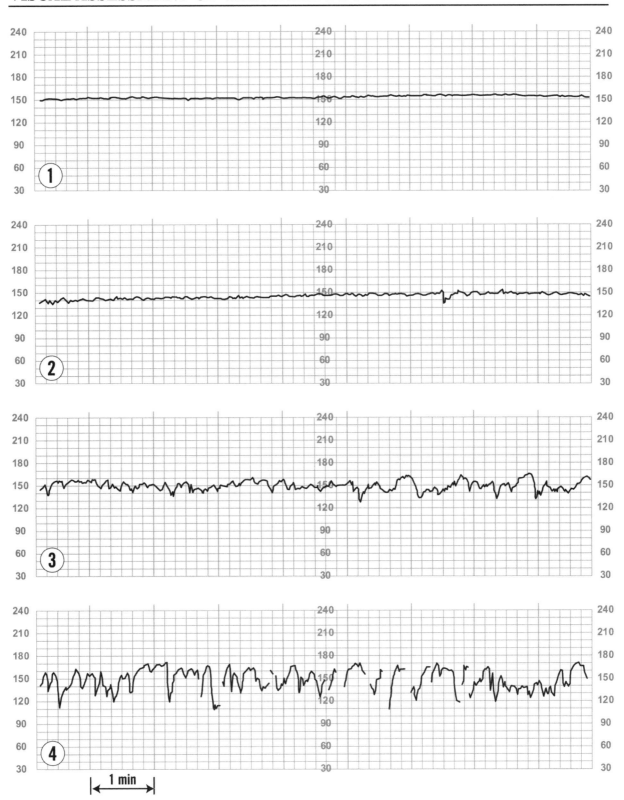

Source: Adapted from Electronic fetal heart monitoring: Research guidelines for interpretation, National Institutes of Child Health and Human Development Research Planning Workshop, 1997, Journal of Obstetric, Gynecologic and Neonatal Nursing, 26(6), 635–640. Copyright © AWHONN.

FETAL HEART RATE CHARACTERISTICS AND PATTERNS: NICHD (1997)

Term	Definition
Baseline Rate	Approximate mean FHR rounded to increments of 5 bpm during a 10-minute segment, excluding periodic or episodic changes, periods of marked variability, and segments of baseline that differs by >25 bpm. In any 10-minute window, the minimum baseline duration must be at least 2 minutes or the baseline for that period is indeterminate. In this case, one may need to refer to the previous 10-minute segment for determination of the baseline.
Bradycardia	Baseline rate of <110 bpm.
Tachycardia	Baseline rate of >160 bpm.
Baseline Variability	Fluctuations in the baseline FHR of 2 cycles per minute or greater. These fluctuations are irregular in amplitude and frequency and are visually quantified as the amplitude of the peak to trough in bpm.
- Absent variability	Amplitude range undetectable.
- Minimal variability	Amplitude range visually detectable (>undetectable) but ≤5 bpm.
- Moderate variability	Amplitude range 6–25 bpm.
- Marked variability	Amplitude range >25 bpm.
Acceleration	Visually apparent *abrupt* increase (onset to peak is < 30 seconds) in FHR above baseline. The increase is calculated from the most recently determined portion of the baseline. Acme is ≥ 15 bpm. above the baseline and lasts ≥ 15 seconds and <2 minutes from the onset to return to baseline. Before 32 weeks of gestation, an acme ≥10 bpm above the baseline and duration of ≥10 seconds is an acceleration.
Prolonged acceleration	Acceleration ≥2 minutes and <10 minutes duration.
Early deceleration	Visually apparent *gradual* decrease (onset to nadir is ≥ 30 seconds) of the FHR and return to baseline associated with a uterine contraction. This decrease is calculated from the most recently determined portion of the baseline. It is coincident in timing, with the nadir of deceleration occurring at the same time as the peak of the contraction. In most cases, the onset, nadir, and recovery of the deceleration are coincident with the beginning, peak, and ending of the contraction, respectively.

(continued)

Late deceleration	Visually apparent *gradual* decrease (onset to nadir is ≥ 30 seconds) of the FHR and return to baseline associated with a uterine contraction. This decrease is calculated from the most recently determined portion of the baseline. It is delayed in timing, with the nadir of deceleration occurring after the peak of the contraction. In most cases, the onset, nadir, and recovery of the deceleration occur after the onset, peak, and ending of the contraction, respectively.
Variable deceleration	Visually apparent *abrupt* decrease (onset to beginning of nadir is <30 seconds) in FHR below baseline. The decrease is calculated from the most recently determined portion of the baseline. Decrease is ≥ 15 bpm, lasting ≥ 15 seconds and <2 minutes from onset to return to baseline. When variable decelerations are associated with uterine contractions, their onset, depth, and duration vary with successive uterine contractions.
Prolonged deceleration	Visually apparent decrease in FHR below baseline. The decrease is calculated from the most recently determined portion of the baseline. Decrease is ≥ 15 bpm, lasting ≥ 2 minutes but <10 minutes from onset to return to baseline.

Source: From the National Institute of Child Health and Human Development Research Planning Workshop: Electronic fetal heart rate monitoring: Research guidelines for interpretation. *American Journal of Obstetrics and Gynecology* (1997) 177(6), 1,385–1,390; and *Journal of Obstetric, Gynecologic and Neonatal Nursing* (1997), 26(6) 635–640.

REFERENCE LIST AND BIBLIOGRAPHY

American College of Obstetricians & Gynecologists (ACOG). (2005a). *Compendium of selected publications.* Washington, DC: Author.

American College of Obstetricians & Gynecologists (ACOG). (2005b). Intrapartum fetal heart rate monitoring. (Practice Bulletin 62). Washington, DC: Author.

American College of Obstetricians & Gynecologists. (ACOG). *Diagnosis and management of preeclampsia and eclampsia* (Practice Bulletin 33). Washington, DC: Author.

American College of Obstetricians & Gynecologists (ACOG). (2003) *Dystocia and augmentation of labor* (Practice Bulletin 49). Washington, DC: Author.

American College of Obstetricians & Gynecologists (ACOG). (2002a). *Antenatal corticosteroid therapy for fetal maturation* (Committee Opinion 273). Washington, DC: Author.

American College of Obstetricians & Gynecologists (ACOG). (2002b). *Prevention of early-onset group B streptococcal disease in newborns* (Committee Opinion 279). Washington, DC: Author.

American College of Obstetricians & Gynecologists (ACOG). (2001a). *Fetal pulse oximetry* (Committee Opinion 258). Washington, DC: Author.

American College of Obstetricians & Gynecologists (ACOG). (2001b). *Prenatal diagnosis of fetal chromosomal abnormalities* (Practice Bulletin 27). Washington, DC: Author.

American College of Obstetricians & Gynecologists (ACOG). (1999a). *Antepartum fetal surveillance* (Practice Bulletin 9). Washington, DC: Author.

American College of Obstetricians & Gynecologists (ACOG). (1999b). *Induction of labor* (Practice Bulletin 10). Washington, DC: Author.

American College of Obstetricians & Gynecologists (ACOG). (1997). *Management of postterm pregnancy* (Practice Patterns 6). Washington, DC: Author.

American College of Obstetricians & Gynecologists (ACOG). (1996). *Assessment of fetal lung maturity* (Technical Bulletin 230). Washington, DC: Author.

American College of Obstetricians & Gynecologists (ACOG). (1994). *Utility of umbilical cord blood acid-base assessment* (Committee Opinion No. 138). Washington, DC: Author.

American Academy of Pediatrics & American College of Obstetricians and Gynecologists. (2002). *Guidelines for perinatal care* (5th ed.). Washington, DC: Authors.

Andres, Saade, Gilstrap, Wilkins, Witline, Zlatnick, & Hankins. (1999). Association between umbilical blood gas parameters and neonatal morbidity and death in neonates with pathologic fetal acidemia. *American Journal of Obstetrics & Gynecology 181:* 867–871.

Arias, F. (1978). Intrauterine resuscitation with terbutaline: A method for management of acute intrapartum fetal distress. *American Journal of Obstetrics and Gynecology, 131*(1), 39–43.

Association of Women's Health, Obstetric and Neonatal Nurses (AWHONN). (2003). *Fetal heart monitoring principles and practices* (3rd ed.). Washington, DC: Author.

Association of Women's Health, Obstetric and Neonatal Nurses (AWHONN). (2000a). *Evidence-based clinical practice guideline: Nursing management of the second stage of labor.* Washington, DC: Author.

Association of Women's Health, Obstetric and Neonatal Nurses (AWHONN). (2000b). *Fetal assessment. Position statement.* Washington, DC: Author.

Association of Women's Health, Obstetric and Neonatal Nurses (AWHONN). (1998). *Clinical competencies and education guide: Fetal surveillance in antepartum and intrapartum nursing practice.* Washington, DC: Author.

Association of Women's Health, Obstetric and Neonatal Nurses (AWHONN). (1997). *Fetal heart monitoring principles and practices* (2nd ed.). Washington, DC: Author.

Barnett, M.M., & Humenick, S.S. (1982). *Infant outcome in relation to second stage labor pushing method. Birth, 9:* 221–229.

Barton, J.R., O'Brien, J.M., Bergauer, N.K., Jacques, D.L., & Sibai, B.M. (2001). *Mild gestational hypertension remote from term: Progression and outcome. American Journal of Obstetrics and Gynecology, 184*(5), 979–983.

Beischer, N.A., Mackay, E.V., & Colditz, P.B. (1997). *Obstetrics and the newborn: An illustrated textbook* (3rd ed.). Philadelphia: W.B. Saunders.

Bishop, E.H. (1981). *Fetal acceleration test. American Journal of Obstetrics and Gynecology, 141*(8), 905–909.

Bochner, C.J., Williams, J., III, Castro, L., Medearis, A., Hobel, C.J., & Wade, M. (1988). The efficacy of starting postterm antenatal testing at 41 weeks as compared with 42 weeks of gestational age. *American Journal of Obstetrics and Gynecology, 159*(3), 550–554.

Brown, C.E. (1998). *Intrapartum tocolysis: An option for acute intrapartum fetal crisis. Journal of Obstetric, Gynecologic, and Neonatal Nursing, 27*(3), 257–261.

Canadian Perinatal Regionalization Coalition, Society of Obstetricians and Gynecologists of Canada, and Provincial Perinatal Education and Outreach Programs (2000). *Fundamentals of fetal health surveillance in labour.* Workshop prereading manual. Author.

Chanraharan, E., & Arulkumaran, S. (2005). *Acute tocolysis. Current Opinion in Obstetrics & Gynecology, 17:* 151–156.

Chua, S., & Arulkumaran, S. (1999). Prolonged pregnancy. In: D.K. James, P.J. Steer, C.R. Weiner, & B. Gonik (Eds.). *High risk pregnancy management options* (2nd ed., pp. 1057–1061) Philadelphia: W.B. Saunders.

Clark, S.L., Cotton, D.B., Pivarnik, J.M., Lee, W., Hankins, G.D., Benedetti, T.J., et al. (1991). Position change and central hemodynamic profile during normal third trimester and post partum. *American Journal of Obstetrics and Gynecology, 164*(3), 883–887.

Crane & Young (1998). Meta-analysis of low-dose versus high-dose oxytocin for labour induction. *Journal of the Society of Obstericians & Gynaecologists of Canada, 20:* 1215–1223.

Creasy, R.K., & Resnik, R. (Eds). (1999). *Maternal-fetal medicine* (4th ed.). Philadelphia: W.B. Saunders.

Cunningham, F. G., Gant, N.F., Leveno, K.J., Gilstrap, L.C., III, Hauth, J.C., & Wenstrom, K.D. (2001). *Williams obstetrics* (21sted.). New York: McGraw-Hill.

Daniel-Spiegel, Weiner, Ben-Shlomo & Shalev (2004). For how long should oxytocin be continued during labor? *BJOG: An International Journal of Obstetrics and Gynecology, 111:* 331–334.

Druzin, M.L., Fox, A., Kogut, E., & Carlson, C. (1985). The relationship of the nonstress test to gestational age. *American Journal of Obstetrics and Gynecology, 153(4),* 386–389.

Eganhouse, D.J., & Burnside, S.M. (1992). Nursing assessment and responsibilities in monitoring the preterm pregnancy. *Journal of Obstetric, Gynecologic and Neonatal Nursing, 21*(5), 355–363.

Feinstein, N.F., Sprague, A., & Trepanier, M.J. (2000). *Fetal heart auscultation.* Washington, DC: Association of Women's Health, Obstetric and Neonatal Nurses.

Fox, M. (2004). Obstetric emergencies. Presented at Synergy: High Risk Obstetric & Neonatal Nursing, November 4 2004. San Francisco, CA.

Fox, M., Kilpatrick, S., King, T., & Parer, J.T. (2000). Fetal heart rate monitoring: Interpretation and collaborative management. *Journal of Nurse Midwifery & Women's Health, 45:* 498–507.

Fraser, W., et al. (2005). Amnioinfusion for the prevention of meconium aspiration syndrome. *New England Journal of Medicine, 353:* 909–917.

Freeman, R.K., Garite, T.J., & Nageotte, M.P. (1991). *Fetal heart rate monitoring* (2nd ed.). Baltimore: Williams & Wilkins.

Gabbe, S.G., Niebyl, J.R. & Simpson, J.L. (Eds.). (2002). *Obstetrics: Normal and problem pregnancies* (4th ed.). New York: Churchill Livingstone.

Garite, T.J. (2002). Intrapartum fetal evaluation. In S.G. Gabbe, J.R. Niebyl, & J.L. Simpson (Eds). *Obstetrics: Normal and problem pregnancies,* pp. 395–429. New York: Churchill Livingstone.

Garite, T.J., & Porreco, R.P. (2001). Evaluating fetal hypoxia with pulse oximetry. *Contemporary OB/GYN, 46*(7), 13–26.

Gilstrap, L.C. (2004). Fetal acid-base balance. In R.K. Creasy, R. Resnick, & J.D. Iams (Eds.), *Maternal-fetal medicine: Principles and practice* (5th ed.), p. 434.

Grannum, P.A., Berkowitz, R.L., & Hobbins, J.C. (1979). The ultrasonic changes in the maturing placenta and their relation to fetal pulmonic maturity. *American Journal of Obstetrics and Gynecology, 133*(8), 915–922.

Hickson, G.B., Federspiel, C.F., Pichert, J.W., Miller, C.S., Gauld-Jaeger, J., & Bost, P. (2002). Patient complaints and malpractice risk. *JAMA, 287:* 2951–2957.

Jauniaux, E., & Campbell, S. (1991). Antenatal diagnosis of placental infarcts by ultrasonography. *Journal of Clinical Ultrasound, 19*(1), 58–61.

JCAHO (2005). 2006 critical access hospital and hospital national patient safety goals. Goal 2E: "Implement a standardized approach to 'hand off' communications, including an opportunity to ask and respond to questions." Accessed August 8, 2005 at www.jcipatientsafety.org/show.asp?durki=10293&site=164&return=10289.

JCAHO. (2004). Focus on five: Strategies for enhancing physician-to-physician and staff-to-physician communication. *Joint Commission Perspectives on Patient Safety, 4*(11).

Keenan, G.M., Cooke, R., & Hillis, S.L. (1998). *Norms and nurse management of conflicts: Keys to understanding nurse-physician collaboration. Research in Nursing and Health, 2,* 59–72.

Klavan, M., Laver, A.L., & Boscola, M.A. (1977). *Clinical concepts of fetal heart rate monitoring.* Waltham, MA: Hewlett-Packard Co.

Krebs, H.B., Petres, R.E., & Dunn, L.J. (1983). Intrapartum fetal heart rate monitoring VIII. Atypical variable deceleration. *American Journal of Obstetrics and Gynecology, 145*(3), 297–305.

Lavin, J.P., Jr., Miodovnik, M., & Barden, T.P. (1984). Relationship of nonstress test reactivity and gestational age. *Obstetrics and Gynecology, 63*(3), 338–344.

Lee, C.Y., Di Loreto, P.C., & O'Lane, J.M. (1975). A study of fetal heart rate acceleration patterns. *Obstetrics and Gynecology, 45*(2), 142–146.

Lindsay, M.K. (1999). Intrauterine resuscitation of the compromised fetus. *Clinics in Perinatology, 26*(3), 569–584.

Liston, R., Crane, J., Hamilton, E., Hughes, O., Kuling, S., MacKinnon, C., et al. (2002a). Clinical practice guideline: Fetal health surveillance in labour. *Journal of the Society of Obstetricians and Gynaecologists of Canada, 24*(3), 250–252.

Liston, R., Crane, J., Hamilton, E., Hughes, O., Kuling, S., MacKinnon, C., et al. (2002b). Clinical practice guideline: Fetal health surveillance in labour. *Journal of the Society of Obstetricians and Gynaecologists of Canada, 24*(4), 342–355.

Low, J.A., Lindsay & Derrick, E.J. (1997). Threshold of metabolic acidosis associated with newborn complications. *American Journal of Obstetrics & Gynecology, 177:* 1391–1394.

Low, J.A., Victory, R., & Derrick, E.J. (1999) Predictive value of electronic fetal monitoring for intrapartum fetal asphyxia with metabolic acidosis, *Obstetrics & Gynecology, 93:* 285–291.

McGee, D.C. (1997). Assessment of fetal lung maturity. *Neonatal Network, 16*(3), 59–63.

Mead, P., Hager, W.D., & Faro, S. (Eds.). (1999). *Protocols for infectious diseases in obstetrics and gynecology* (2nd ed.). Oxford, UK: Blackwell Science Inc.

Menihan, C., & Zottoli, E.K. (2001). *Electronic fetal monitoring: Concepts and applications.* Philadelphia: Lippincott.

Murray, M. (1997). *Antepartal and intrapartal fetal monitoring.* Albuquerque, NM: Learning Resources International, Inc.

National Institute of Child Health and Human Development Research Planning Workshop (1997). Electronic fetal heart rate monitoring: Research guidelines for interpretation. *Journal of Obstetric, Gynecologic and Neonatal Nursing 26*(6), 635–640.

National Institute of Child Health and Human Development Research Planning Workshop (1998). Electronic fetal heart rate monitoring: Research guidelines for interpretation. *American Journal of Obstetrics and Gynecology, 177*(6) 1385–1390.

National Institutes of Health. (2000a). *Antenatal corticosteroids revisited: Repeat courses.* Washington, DC: Author.

National Institutes of Health. (2000b). Report of the National High Blood Pressure Education Program Working Group on High Blood Pressure in Pregnancy. *American Journal of Obstetrics and Gynecology, 183:* S1–S22.

O'Grady, J.P., Parker, R.K., & Patel, S.S. (2000). Nitroglycerine for rapid tocolysis: Development of a protocol and a literature review. *Journal of Perinatology, 1:* 27–33.

Parer, J.T. (1983). *Handbook of fetal heart rate monitoring.* Philadelphia: W.B. Saunders.

Parer, J.T. (1997). *Handbook of fetal heart rate monitoring* (2nd ed.). Philadelphia: W.B. Saunders.

Patriarco, M.S., Viechnicki, B.M., Hutchinson, T.A., Klasko, S.K., & Yeh, S.Y. (1987). A study on intrauterine resuscitation with terbutaline. *American Journal of Obstetrics and Gynecology, 157*(2), 384–387.

Phaneuf, Rodrigues Linares, TambyRaja, MacKenzie, & Lopez Bernal. (2000). Loss of myometrial oxytocin receptors during oxytocin-induced and oxytocin-augmented labour. *Journal of Reproduction and Fertility, 120:* 91–97.

Porter, M.L. (2000). Fetal pulse oximetry: An adjunct to electronic fetal heart rate monitoring. *Journal of Obstetric, Gynecologic, and Neonatal Nursing, 29*(5), 537-548.

Roberts, J. (2002). The "push" for evidence: Management of the second stage. *Journal of Midwifery & Women's Health,47:*2–15

Rommal, C. (1996). Risk management issues in the perinatal setting. *Journal of Perinatal and Neonatal Nursing, 10*(3), 1–31.

Rouse, Owen, Savage, & Hauth. (2001). Active phase labor arrest: Revisiting the two hour minimum. *Obstetrics & Gynecology, 98:* 550–554.

Sarno, A.P., Jr., & Phelan, J.P. (1988). Intrauterine resuscitation of the fetus. *Contemporary OB/GYN, 31*(7), 143–152.

Simpson, K.R. (2005). Perinatal patient safety: Handling handoffs safely. *MCN: The American Journal of Maternal-Child Nursing, 30:* 152.

Simpson, K.R. (2002). *Cervical ripening and induction and augmentation of Labor* (2nd ed.). Washington, DC: Association of Women's Health, Obstetric and Neonatal Nurses.

Simpson, K.R. (1998). Intrapartum fetal oxygen saturation monitoring: Ongoing clinical research explores partnering new method with EFM. *AWHONN Lifelines, 2*(6), 20–24.

Simpson, K.R., & Creehan, P.A. (Eds.). (2001a). *Perinatal nursing* (2nd ed.). Philadelphia: Lippincott.

Simpson, K.R., & Chez, B.F. (2001b). Professional and legal issues. In K. Simpson & P. Creehan (Eds). *Perinatal nursing* (2nd ed., pp. 21-52). Philadelphia: Lippincott.

Simpson, K.R., & James. (2005a) Effects of immediate versus delayed pushing during second stage labor on fetal well-being, *Nursing Research, 54*(3): 140–157.

Simpson, K.R., & James. (2005b). Efficacy of intrauterine resuscitation techniques in improving fetal oxygen status during labor. *Obstetrics & Gynecology, 105:* 1362–1368.

Simpson, K.R., & Knox, G.E. (2003). Adverse perinatal outcomes: Recognizing, understanding, and preventing common types of accidents. *AWHONN Lifelines, 7,* 224–235.

Simpson, K.R., & Knox, G. (2001). Strategies for developing an evidence-based approach to perinatal care. *MCN: American Journal of Maternal Child Nursing, 24*(3), 122–132.

Simpson, K.R., & Porter, M.L. (2001). Fetal oxygen saturation monitoring: Using this new technology for fetal assessment during labor. *AWHONN Lifelines, 5*(2), 26–33.

Society of Obstetricians and Gynaecologists of Canada. (1995). Fetal health surveillance in labour (policy statement). *Journal of the Society of Obstetricians and Gynaecologists of Canada, 17*(9), 865–901.

Steutel, M. (2000). Intrapartum nursing care: A case study of supportive interventions and ethical conflicts. *Birth: Issues in Perinatal Care, 27*(1), 38–45.

Thorp, J.A., & Rushing, R.S. (1999). Umbilical cord blood analysis. *Obstetrics and Gynecology Clinics of North America, 26*(4), 695–711.

Tucker, S.M. (2000). *Fetal monitoring and assessment* (4th ed.). St Louis: Mosby.

Von Oech, R. (1983). *A whack on the side of the head: How you can be more creative.* New York: Warner Books.

Williams, K.P., & Galerneau, F. (2003) Intrapartum fetal heart rate patterns in the prediction of neonatal acidemia. *American Journal of Obstetrics & Gynecology, 188:* 820–823.

Yeomans, E.R., Hauth, J.C., Gilstrap, L.C., III, & Strickland, D.M. (1985). Umbilical cord pH, pCO and bicarbonate following uncomplicated term vaginal deliveries. *American Journal of Obstetrics and Gynecology, 151*(6), 798–800.

Young, B. (1990). Placental regulation of fetal oxygenation and acid-base balance. In R.D. Eden & F.H. Boehm (Eds.), *Assessment and care of the fetus, physiological, clinical, and medicalegal principles* (Chap. 11, pp. 171–177). Norwalk, CT: Appleton and Lange.

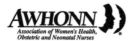

Association of Women's Health, Obstetric and Neonatal Nurses

AWHONN Membership Application

RECRUITED BY   (IF APPLICABLE):   RECRUITER'S MEMBER #:

Membership categories (Choose one)

☐ **Full $149**
RNs licensed in the US, its territories or Canada. May hold elected and appointed offices and may vote.

☐ **Associate $132**
LPNs, LVNs or others interested in the health of women and newborns. May hold appointed office, but may not vote.

☐ **Student $75**
Eligible for 4 years. RNs may vote. Proof of current enrollment required. Please attach.

☐ **Retired $75**
Must be at least 62 and no longer working as a nurse. Min. 3 years previous full membership required. RNs may vote.

☐ **Disabled $75**
Unable to work. Statement by applicant is acceptable. RNs may vote.

☐ **International $173**
A nurse or oth er interested party residing outside the US (other than members of the US Armed Forces). RNs may vote.

PREFIX (MS, MR, ETC)   FIRST   MI   LAST   SUFFIX (JR., III, ETC)

CREDENTIALS (RN, CNM, ETC)   TITLE/POSITION (E.G. NURSE MANAGER, MIDWIFE, DIRECTOR, ETC)

HOME ADDRESS   CITY   STATE/PROVINCE

ZIP/POSTAL CODE   COUNTRY   HOME PHONE

EMPLOYER   WORK ADDRESS   CI TY   STATE/PROVINCE   ZIP/POSTAL CODE

WORK PHONE   WORK FAX

PREFERRED E-MAIL ADDRESS FOR AWHONN COMMUNICATION

PREFERRED MAILING ADDRESS (CHECK ONE)   ☐ WORK   ☐ HOME

☐ I AM CURRENTLY AN ACTIVE DUTY MEMBER OF THE US ARMED FORCES. BRANCH OF SERVICE (CHECK ONE)   ☐ ARMY   ☐ NAVY   ☐ AIR FORCE
   (ACTIVE DUTY MEMBERS OF THE US ARMED FORCES WILL BE MEMBERS OF THE AWHONN ARMED FORCES SECTION.)
   RANK :

☐ I AM AFFILIATED WITH THE US ARMED FORCES (RETIRED, RESERVIST, DOD CIVILIAN, ETC) BUT AM NOT ON ACTIVE DUTY, AND I WOULD LIKE TO BE A MEMBER
   OF THE AWHONN ARMED FORCES SECTION INSTEAD OF THE SECTION IN WHICH I RESIDE.

WE OCCASIONALLY MAKE OUR MAILING LIST AVAILABLE TO CAREFULLY SCREENED ORGANIZATIONS THAT OFFER PRODUCTS AND/OR SERVICES THAT MAY BE OF
INTEREST TO YOU. ☐ CHECK THIS BOX ONLY IF YOU DO NOT WANT TO RECEIVE SUCH MAILINGS.

Method of Payment   Amount Enclosed

☐ CHECK OR MONEY ORDER PAYABLE TO AWHONN   DUES $

☐ VISA   ☐ MASTERCARD   ☐ AMERICAN EXPRESS   ☐ OPTIONAL TAX-DEDUCTIBLE DONATION TO AWHONN   HEALTHFUNDS $20.00

                                                      TOTAL E NCLOSED $
CARD N O   EXP DATE
                                                      ENTER PROMOTI ON CODE HERE, IF ANY
CARD HO LDE R'S NAME

                                                      SUBMIT APPLICATION AND PAYMENT TO:
SIGNA TURE   AWHONN, Dept. 4015, Washington, DC 20042-4015

                                                      Phone: 800-673-8499; 800-245-0231 (Canada)
*DUES SUBJECT TO CHANGE. MEMBERSHIP DUES ARE NOT REFUNDABLE.   Fax: 202-728-0575; www.awhonn.org

Member Profile

We want to make that sure we offer the professional nursing programs, services and products that are of greatest value to you. Please complete this member profile. Your answers will be kept confidential.

IN NURSING PRACTICE SINCE _____
YEAR ONLY

DATE OF BIRTH _____
DAY MO YR

GENDER   ☐ M   ☐ F

Primary Position (select no more than 2)
☐ CASE MANAGER
☐ CLINICAL NURSE SPECIALIST
☐ CONSULTANT
☐ FACULTY-ACADEMIC
☐ NURSE EXECUTIVE
☐ NURSE MANAGER/COORDINATOR
☐ NURSE MIDWIFE
☐ NURSE PRACTITIONER
☐ RESEARCHER
☐ STAFF DEVELOPMENT
☐ STAFF NURSE
☐ STUDENT
☐ OTHER: _____

Ethnic/Racial Background (select one)
☐ AMERICAN INDIAN/ALASKA NATIVE
☐ ASIAN OR PACIFIC ISLANDER
☐ AFRICAN AMERICAN (NON-HISPANIC)
☐ HISPANIC
☐ WHITE (NON-HISPANIC)
☐ MULTIRACIAL

Certifications (check all that apply)
☐ AMBULATORY WOMEN'S HEALTH
☐ CHILDBIRTH EDUCATOR
☐ EFM/FHM
☐ HIGH-RISK OB NURSING
☐ INPATIENT OB
☐ LACTATION CONSULTANT/EDUCATOR
☐ LOW-RISK NEONATAL NURSING
☐ MATERNAL NEWBORN NURSING
☐ NICU NURSING
☐ NEONATAL NURSE PRACTITIONER
☐ NURSING ADMINISTRATION
☐ NURSE MIDWIFE
☐ OB/GYN PRACTITIONER
☐ PERINATAL NURSE PRACTITIONER
☐ PERINATAL NURSING
☐ WOMEN'S HEALTH NURSE PRACTIONER
☐ OTHER: _____

Highest Degree Earned
☐ DOCTORATE
☐ MASTER'S
☐ BACHELOR'S
☐ ASSOCIATE
☐ DIPLOMA
☐ VOC-TECH
☐ OTHER: _____

Medications and/or OTC Products (check all that apply)
☐ HAVE PRESCRIPTIVE AUTHORITY
☐ RECOMMEND MEDICATION AND/OR OTC PRODUCTS
☐ COUNSEL AND EDUCATE PATIENTS REGARDING USE OF MEDICATIONS AND/OR OTC PRODUCTS
☐ NO ROLE REGARDING MEDICATIONS AND/OR OTC PRODUCTS

Equipment and Supplies (check all that apply)
☐ MAKE PURCHASING DECISIONS DIRECTLY
☐ RECOMMEND OR INFLUENCE DECISIONS
☐ NO ROLE REGARDING PURCHASE OF EQUIPMENT AND/OR SUPPLIES

Primary Clinical Focus (select no more than 2)
☐ ANTEPARTUM
☐ BREASTFEEDING/LACTATION
☐ INTRAPARTUM (INCLUDES LDR/LDRP & L&D)
☐ NICU
☐ NURSERY
☐ WOMEN'S HEALTH
☐ POSTPARTUM (INCLUDES MOTHER-BABY)
☐ OTHER: _____

Job Setting
☐ ACADEMIA
☐ AMBULATORY CARE (INCLUDES PHYSICIAN OFFICE, OUTPATIENT CLINIC, ETC.)
☐ HOME HEALTH CARE
☐ HOSPITAL INPATIENT
☐ NOT WORKING
☐ PUBLIC HEALTH
☐ SELF-EMPLOYED
☐ OTHER: _____

Majority of Time Spent (select no more than 2)
☐ ADMINISTRATION
☐ CONSULTING
☐ DIRECT PATIENT CARE
☐ MANAGEMENT/SUPERVISION
☐ PATIENT EDUCATION
☐ RESEARCH
☐ STAFF DEVELOPMENT/EDUCATION
☐ UNDERGRAD/GRADUATE NURSING EDUCATION
☐ OTHER: _____

Is Continuing Education (CE) required for you to maintain licensure and/or certification?
☐ YES   ☐ NO

Other memberships
☐ AACN (CRITICAL CARE NURSES)   ☐ AANP   ☐ ACNM   ☐ ANA
☐ ANN   ☐ AONE   ☐ NANN   ☐ NPWH   ☐ SIGMA THETA TAU
☐ OTHER: _____

How did you learn about AWHONN?
☐ COLLEAGUE
☐ ADVERTISEMENT
☐ MAILING
☐ CONFERENCE/CONVENTION
☐ OTHER: _____

SUBMIT APPLICATION AND PAYMENT TO:
AWHONN, Dept. 4015, Washington, DC 20042-4015

Phone: 800-673-8499; 800-245-0231 (Canada)
Fax: 202-728-0575; www.awhonn.org

COURSE OUTLINE

Intermediate
Fetal Monitoring Course

©2006 AWHONN

Course Objectives

1. Analyze fetal heart rate patterns, uterine activity and their implications for fetal well-being.

2. Correlate indicated clinical interventions with related maternal-fetal physiology.

3. Effectively communicate verbal and written data about patient status.

4. Describe the roles and responsibilities of health care providers in the use of FHM in intrapartum care.

5. Demonstrate the decision-making process necessary for the proper selection and verification of fetal heart monitoring (FHM) techniques.

6. Simulate the psychomotor skills used in FHM.

2 ©2006 AWHONN

Transition to NICHD Definitions

All of the AWHONN Fetal Heart Monitoring Program (FHMP) components now include the NICHD fetal heart monitoring definitions presented in the original 1997 articles published simultaneously in:

■ *Journal of Obstetric, Gynecologic and Neonatal Nursing (JOGNN)*

■ *American Journal of Obstetrics and Gynecology*

3 ©2006 AWHONN

Why Transition to NICHD?

- Standardization and simplification of key clinical terms and protocols are fundamental principles of patient safety.
- Standardized terminology for fetal monitoring was recommended by JCAHO in the July 2004 Sentinel Event Alert #30
- Use of consistent FHM terminology among professional associations is optimal.

4 ©2006 AWHONN

Root Causes of Perinatal Deaths and Injuries
JCAHO 1995 - 2004

Communication
Orientation/training
Patient assessment
Staffing
Availability of info
Competency/credentialing
Procedural compliance
Environ. safety/security
Leadership
Continuum of care
Care planning
Organization culture

Includes issues related to accurate interpretation and timely communication of fetal assessment data

0 10 20 30 40 50 60 70 80 90 100

(Joint Commission on Accreditation of Healthcare Organizations [JCAHO], 2004)

5 ©2006 AWHONN

Potential Benefits: One Language

- Everyone on the perinatal team speaking the same language when communicating about fetal assessment data
- Clear concise terms to minimize variations among providers
- Consistency in medical record documentation of fetal status
- Decreased liability exposure

6 ©2006 AWHONN

Visual Determination of FHR Patterns

- Primarily developed for visual interpretation
- Mathematical quantification of definitions are general guidelines
- Quantitative and qualitative interpretation
- "In most cases", "approximate" are terms included in definitions

7 ©2006 AWHONN

Visual Determination of FHR Patterns

- The definitions apply to the interpretation of FHR patterns produced from either a direct fetal electrode detecting the fetal electrocardiogram or an external Doppler device detecting the fetal heart events with use of the autocorrelation technique.
- Assuming a readable tracing is obtained, there is no inherent need for amniotomy, spiral electrode and/or intrauterine pressure catheter insertion for FHR pattern interpretation.

8 ©2006 AWHONN

Primary Differences: NICHD and Former AWHONN Terminology

- Baseline rounded to increments of 5 bpm during a 10-minute segment (e.g., 135, 140, 145, 150, etc.)
- Baseline determined between periodic or episodic changes (no mention of between contractions)
- Elimination of the distinction between short-term variability and long-term variability
- Slight differences in terms and ranges for variability

9 ©2006 AWHONN

periodic = c̄ ctx
episodic s̄ relation to ctx

Primary Differences (Cont.)

- One type of variable deceleration (elimination of the need to include atypical characteristics when identifying a variable deceleration)
- Elimination of combination deceleration patterns (acknowledgement that two or more types of decelerations may occur within a 10-min. segment)
- The term *nonperiodic* changed to *episodic*
- The term *persistent* changed to *recurrent* (decelerations occurring with ≥ 50% of contractions within a 20-min. segment)

10 ©2006 AWHONN

Determination and Documentation of Baseline Rate

- Baseline FHR is the approximate mean FHR rounded to increments of 5 bpm during a 10-min. segment excluding:
  - › Periodic or episodic (previously known as *nonperiodic*) changes
  - › Periods of marked FHR variability
  - › Segments of baseline that differ by >25 bpm
- Baseline can be determined between contractions.
- Rate plus baseline variability give the indication of range (e.g., a baseline of 145 bpm with moderate variability indicates a range of 6 to 25 bpm).

11 ©2006 AWHONN

Periodic and Episodic Patterns

- Accelerations and decelerations are categorized as either periodic or episodic.
- Periodic patterns are those associated with uterine contractions.
- Episodic patterns are those not associated with uterine contractions. (The FHMP has previously used the term *nonperiodic* rather than episodic).

12 ©2006 AWHONN

Baseline Variability

- No distinction is made between short-term variability (or beat-to-beat variability or R-R wave period differences in the electrocardiogram) and long-term variability because in actual practice they are visually determined as a unit.

- Hence, the definition of variability is based visually on the amplitude of the complexes, with exclusion of the regular, smooth sinusoidal pattern.

13 ©2006 AWHONN

Baseline Variability

Undetectable from baseline Absent	
Visually detectable from baseline, but ≤ 5 bpm Minimal	
6 – 25 bpm Moderate	
> 25 bpm Marked	

14 ©2006 AWHONN

Variable Decelerations

- Variable decelerations are inherently variable in timing, shape and duration.

- Physiologic implications and appropriate interventions are the same for all variable decelerations considering the baseline variability, clinical context, and how long the pattern has been evolving.

- There is no need to further describe each variable deceleration by atypical features.

15 ©2006 AWHONN

Combination Decelerations

- Not all FHR patterns will meet the mathematical criteria in the NICHD definitions exactly.

- Choose the *one* definition that most closely approximates the FHR pattern displayed.

- Terms such as "late variable decelerations", "variable decelerations with a late component", or "variable in shape, but late in timing" are inconsistent with NICHD definitions.

- Some 10- to 20-min. segments may have two or more types of decelerations; identify each type of deceleration appropriately.

16 ©2006 AWHONN

Persistent vs. Recurrent

- Decelerations are defined as recurrent if they occur with ≥ 50% of uterine contractions in any 20-min. segment

- Persistent has been used in the past to describe repetitive FHR patterns but has not been precisely defined

- In some cases, persistency has been defined as usually occurring with ≥ 50% of contractions without a time frame (i.e. 20 min. segment)

17 ©2006 AWHONN

AWHONN))
Association of Women's Health,
Obstetric and Neonatal Nurses

Assessment

Maternal and Fetal Data Base

©2006 AWHONN

Assessment: Maternal Data Base

- History
  - Family
  - Medical/surgical
  - Obstetric
  - Psychosocial issues
- Current Pregnancy
  - Medical/surgical history
  - Obstetric issues
  - Psychosocial issues

19 ©2006 AWHONN

Current Pregnancy

- Prenatal Records
  - Labs
  - Weight gain/loss
  - Vital sign trends
  - Ultrasound reports
  - Fundal height trends
- Patient Interview

20 ©2006 AWHONN

Current Pregnancy

- Physical Assessment
  - Maternal vital signs
  - Oxygenation of maternal-fetal unit
  - Assessment of labor status (maternal)
  - Assessment of labor tolerance:
    - Maternal
    - Fetal

21 ©2006 AWHONN

Tissues - prior birth trauma, sexual abuse
SA, housing issues

Cheryl, 35 years old
G2, P1001, 41 6/7 Weeks Gestation

- History
  - One spontaneous vaginal birth 8 years ago of a healthy 7 lbs., 4 oz. (3,288 gm) full-term male
- Family history
  - Both parents hypertensive

22 ©2006 AWHONN

Cheryl (Cont.)

- Current pregnancy
  - First pregnancy with current partner
  - 10 prenatal visits
  - 47 lbs. (21.3 kg) weight gain
  - Fetal heart rate (FHR) and fetal movements within normal range throughout pregnancy

23 ©2006 AWHONN

Cheryl (Cont.)

Estimated Gestational Age	Blood Pressure
11 weeks: 1st visit	120/76
26 weeks: 4th visit	124/84
35 weeks: 6th visit	140/88
37 weeks: 8th visit	136/86
40 weeks: 10th visit	130/88

24 ©2006 AWHONN

Cheryl (Cont.)

- 18-week Level II ultrasound confirmed dates by LMP and normal anatomy
- Fundal height exams consistent with EDC
- Triple screen (AFP, hCG, E3) within normal limits (WNL)
- Declined amniocentesis
- 2nd trimester glucose screen negative

25 ©2006 AWHONN

Cheryl (Cont.)

- Admission
  - 41 6/7 weeks gestation admitted at 0500
  - Missed 41 week appointment
  - Vaginal exam: 2 cm/70%/-2
  - Fetus vertex by Leopold's maneuvers and vaginal exam
  - Membranes intact, bloody show observed
  - Contractions: q 3-5 min. x 40-50 sec.; moderate by palpation

26 ©2006 AWHONN

Cheryl (Cont.)

- Admission (cont.)
  - Vital signs: BP 140/92, P 92, R 20, T 98° F (36.7° C)
  - Pain score 3/10
  - 3+ pretibial edema
  - 3+ patellar reflexes
  - Denies headache, blurred vision, scotoma, epigastric pain
  - Unable to void

27 ©2006 AWHONN

Systematic Assessment of FHR Tracings

- Baseline rate
- Variability
- Periodic/episodic changes
- Uterine activity
- Pattern evolution
- Accompanying clinical characteristics
- Urgency

(Adapted from Fox, Kilpatrick, King & Parer, 2000)

28 ©2006 AWHONN

Variability – NICHD Terminology

Amplitude of FHR Change	Former AWHONN Baseline LTV Description	NICHD Baseline Variability Description
Undetectable from baseline	Decreased/ Minimal	Absent
Visually detectable from baseline, ≤ 5 bpm	Decreased/Minimal	Minimal
6 – 25 bpm	Average/Within Normal Limits	Moderate
> 25 bpm	Marked/Saltatory	Marked

29 ©2006 AWHONN

Decelerations – NICHD Terminology

Type	Definition: Visually apparent decrease in FHR
Early	*Gradual* onset: ≥ 30 sec from onset to nadir; nadir simultaneous with peak of contraction
Late	*Gradual* onset: ≥ 30 sec from onset to nadir; delayed in timing – nadir after peak of contraction
Variable	*Abrupt* onset: < 30 sec from onset to nadir, lasting ≥ 15 sec but < 2 min.; depth ≥ 15 bpm
Prolonged	Decrease of ≥ 15 bpm lasting ≥ 2 min. but less than 10 minutes (≥ 10 min. = baseline change)

30 ©2006 AWHONN

Cheryl: Admission Tracing

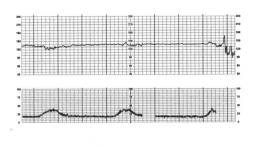

31 ©2006 AWHONN

Chart:
EFM adjusted to ↑ quality of
tracing

Pertinent Historical Data: Hypertension (HTN)

Risks

- Maternal age
- First pregnancy with partner
- Family history of HTN

Signs and Symptoms

- Prenatal BP trends
- Weight gain
- Edema
- 3+ reflexes

32 ©2006 AWHONN

Cheryl: Risk Factors

- Preeclampsia
- Chronic hypertension
- Decreased uterine blood flow
- Decreased kidney function
- Altered neurologic function
- Impaired liver function

33 ©2006 AWHONN

Pertinent Historical Data:
Postdates

- 8-year interval between pregnancies
- Estimated gestational age: 41 6/7 weeks

34 ©2006 AWHONN

Extrinsic Influences on
Fetal Heart Patterns

- Maternal
- Utero-placental perfusion
- Umbilical circulation
- Amniotic fluid characteristics

35 ©2006 AWHONN

Placental Anatomy

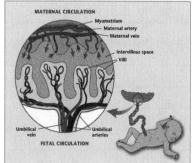

36 ©2006 AWHONN

Placental Aging: Calcification

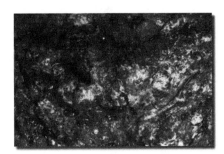

37 ©2006 AWHONN

uterine bloodflow   A
placental function   B
umbilical bloodflow   C

echolucent lesions-lakes
infarctions may be significant -
result from disruption of mat. blood
supply to placenta

Placental Grading

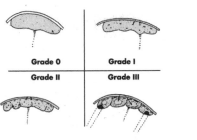

Grade 0   Grade I
Grade II   Grade III

Reprinted from the *American Journal of Obstetrics and Gynecology*, 133(8), by P. A. Grannum, R. L. Berkowitz, and J. C. Hobbins, "The ultrasonic changes in the maturing placenta and their relation to fetal pulmonic maturity", p. 916, © 1979, with permission from Elsevier Science.

38 ©2006 AWHONN

0: immature - 12 wks
1: 30 - 32 wks ← most of preg
2: calcifications + indentations
III: "Swiss cheese"
IV: C/S

Amniotic Fluid Volume (ml)

Weeks Gestation

39 ©2006 AWHONN

Extrinsic Influences: Placental Changes

- Hypertension
  - ➤ Vasoconstriction
  - ➤ Infarcts
- Post-maturity
  - ➤ Degenerative lesions (calcifications or infarcts)
  - ➤ Decreased amniotic fluid volume

40 ©2006 AWHONN

Inside baby

Intrinsic Influences on FHR: Fetal Reserve

- Placental transfer capacity
- Fetal homeostatic compensatory mechanisms

41 ©2006 AWHONN

Placental Integrity Zone

Placental transfer capacity

Placental reserves

Limit of optimum O_2 and CO_2 exchange

"Safety factor" | Poor nutrient transfer of large molecules | Poor O_2 and CO_2 transfer

Normal | Fetal Malnutrition | Placental Respiratory Failure

100% | 75% | 50% | 0%

Adapted from *Handbook of Fetal Heart Rate Monitoring*, J.T. Parer, p. 30, ©1983, with permission from Elsevier Science.

42 ©2006 AWHONN

Fetal Well-Being

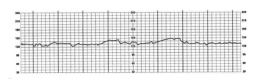

43 ©2006 AWHONN

Post-Term Pregnancy
with Nonreactive Nonstress Test

Potential observations:

- Decreased amniotic fluid index
- Decelerations of the fetal heart rate in labor
- Lower Apgar scores
- Increased need for neonatal resuscitation
- Increased neonatal morbidity

44 ©2006 AWHONN

Post-Term Surveillance

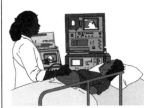

- Nonstress test twice/week
- Amniotic fluid volume twice/week
- Daily fetal movement counts

45 ©2006 AWHONN

Fetal Homeostatic Compensatory Mechanisms

Ability of the fetus to maintain homeostasis when physiologically stressed

pretem - ↓ well developed comp. mec
term may have placenta c̄
small, ↓ blood flow

Uterine Contractions: Effects on Fetus

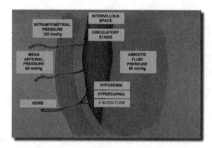

Fetal Circulation

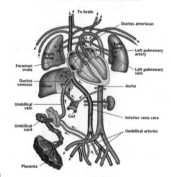

Fetal Responses

- Autonomic nervous system
- Baroreceptors
- Chemoreceptors
- Hormonal responses

49 ©2006 AWHONN

Intrinsic Influences on the FHR

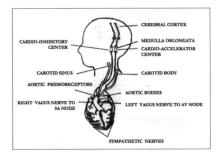

50 ©2006 AWHONN

Fetal Response to Stressors

Hypoxemia and/or decreased umbilical blood flow
↓
Chemoreceptor/baroreceptor stimulation
↓
Catecholamine production
↓
↓ Blood flow to periphery (gastrointestinal and renal)
↓
↑ Blood flow to vital organs (brain, heart, and adrenal)
↓
FHR Changes
(Type of FHR change depends upon nature
and timing of the stressor)

51 ©2006 AWHONN

Blood Redistribution During Fetal Hypoxemia

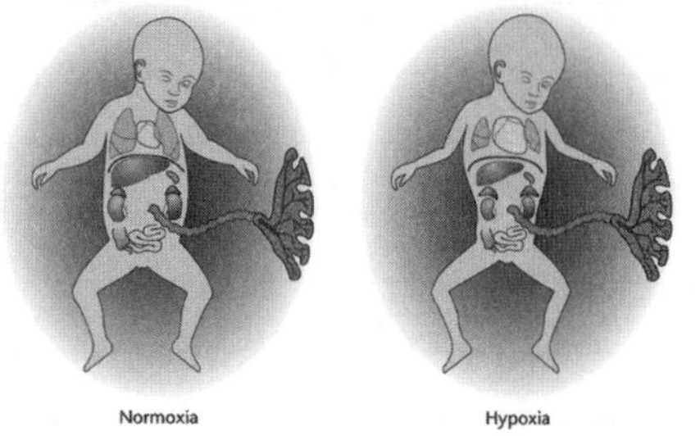

Normoxia   Hypoxia

52 ©2006 AWHONN

Handwritten note: Normoxic

Insufficient placental circulation

+

↓ Blood flow to uterus during contractions

↓ Fetal resources

↑ Risk of fetal compromise

53 ©2006 AWHONN

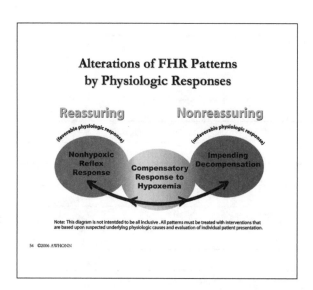

Alterations of FHR Patterns by Physiologic Responses

Reassuring (favorable physiologic response)   **Nonreassuring** (unfavorable physiologic response)

Nonhypoxic Reflex Response — Compensatory Response to Hypoxemia — Impending Decompensation

Note: This diagram is not intentded to be all inclusive. All patterns must be treated with interventions that are based upon suspected underlying physiologic causes and evaluation of individual patient presentation.

54 ©2006 AWHONN

Handwritten note:

mod. variability c̄) compens
recurrent decel

↓ variability c̄ recurrent
decel → impending
decomp

Maternal-Fetal Database

- Risk factors
  - History
  - Current pregnancy
- Physiologic significance
- Implications for fetal well-being

55 ©2006 AWHONN

Maternal and Fetal Physical Assessment

- Maternal vital signs and physical exam
- Fetal presentation
- Fetal movement
- Fetal heart assessment
- Uterine activity
- Labor progress

56 ©2006 AWHONN

The Nursing Process and Fetal Monitoring

ASSESSMENT
Maternal - fetal status, prenatal - perinatal factors, fetal monitoring data

INTERPRETATION
History and review of FHR characteristics

DIAGNOSIS
Patient problems identified independently and collaboratively

EVALUATION
Effects of management on maternal - fetal status; ongoing - FHR/ uterine activity (UA) evaluation; evaluation of interventions

INTERVENTIONS
Independent and collaborative intervention, plan, and implementation

COLLABORATION
Medical Diagnosis, Management & Intervention

Nursing Diagnosis, Management & Intervention

57 ©2006 AWHONN

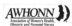

Interpretation

©2006 AWHONN

Exercise:
Five figures are shown below. Select the one that is different from all the others.

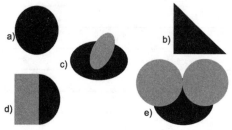

a)

c)

b)

d)

e)

From A WHACK ON THE SIDE OF THE HEAD by Roger von Oech. Copyright ©1983 by
Roger von Oech. By permission of Warner Books, Inc. Reprinted with permission.

59   ©2006 AWHONN

Handwritten notes:

ID events
Support rationale c̄ objective data
not one "right answer"

Helga: Admission History

- Family medical history: Unremarkable
- Medical history: Allergy-related asthma
- Previous pregnancies:
  - Spontaneous abortion (SAB) at 6 weeks
  - 40-week spontaneous vaginal birth of 9 lbs., 1 oz (4110 gm) girl
  - Postpartum depression X 2 weeks after birth

60   ©2006 AWHONN

Helga: Admission History (Cont.)

Current Pregnancy

- Routine prenatal care
- Prenatal labs within normal limits
- 29 lbs. (13.2 kg) weight gain
- Admitted in labor at 5 cm/80%/-1

61 ©2006 AWHONN

Helga (Cont.): Admission Tracing

62 ©2006 AWHONN

Intrinsic Influences on the FHR

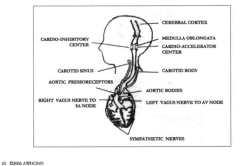

CEREBRAL CORTEX

CARDIO-INHIBITORY CENTER

MEDULLA OBLONGATA

CARDIO-ACCELERATOR CENTER

CAROTID SINUS

CAROTID BODY

AORTIC PRESSORECEPTORS

RIGHT VAGUS NERVE TO SA NODE

AORTIC BODIES

LEFT VAGUS NERVE TO AV NODE

SYMPATHETIC NERVES

63 ©2006 AWHONN

---

baseline 135, mod. variability + accels
Ø decels
reassuring tracing
toco needs adjustment

moderate   strongly associated
variability is a reflection of
adequate fetal cerebral
oxygenation

variability gradually ↓'s

presence of decels = stress
but does not = decompensation
or deoxygenation

Look at evolution of FHR
over time

fetal sleep   } not r/t
arrythmias   } oxygenation
opiods
anomalies
substances

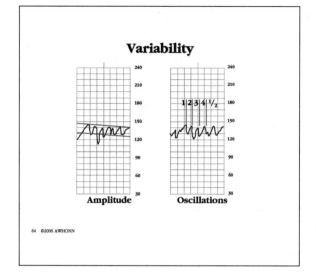

Variability

Amplitude   Oscillations

64 ©2006 AWHONN

Variability

Oscillations

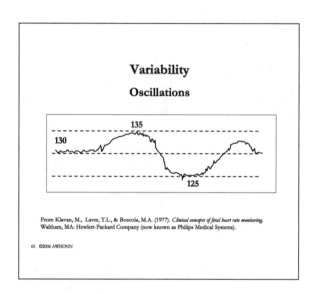

From Klavan, M., Laver, T.L., & Boscola, M.A. (1977). *Clinical concepts of fetal heart rate monitoring.* Waltham, MA: Hewlett-Packard Company (now known as Philips Medical Systems).

65 ©2006 AWHONN

Fetal Heart Rate Range

Amplitude

Range = 10 bpm

From Klavan, M., Laver, T.L., & Boscola, M.A. (1977). *Clinical concepts of fetal heart rate monitoring.* Waltham, MA: Hewlett-Packard Company (now known as Philips Medical Systems).

66 ©2006 AWHONN

Oscillations:
rise + fall within
the baseline range

in 1 min usually 1-6

amplitude:
range or band height
of oscillations
(1-5, 6-25 bpm)

NICHD terminology

variability is one entity;
encompasses long + ST variability

Fetal Heart Rate Variability

Absent	Undectable amplitude
Minimal	Visually dectectable but ≤ 5 bpm amplitude
Moderate	6 - 25 bpm amplitude
Marked	> 25 bpm amplitude

67 ©2006 AWHONN

Moderate Variability

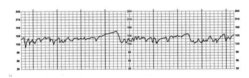

68 ©2006 AWHONN

Absent Variability

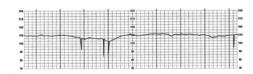

69 ©2006 AWHONN

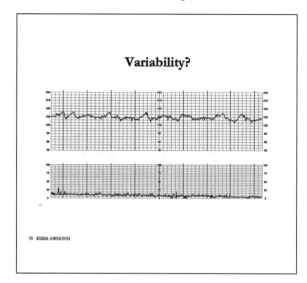

Variability?

70 ©2006 AWHONN

moderate

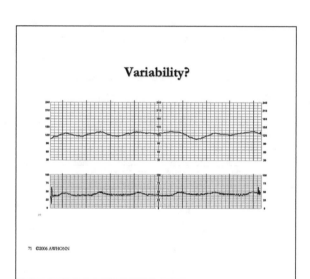

Variability?

71 ©2006 AWHONN

minimal

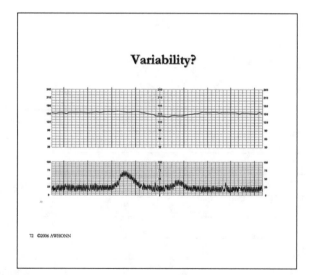

Variability?

72 ©2006 AWHONN

absent

FHR Auscultation

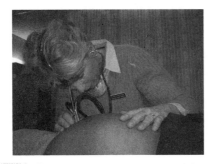

73 ©2006 AWHONN

listen between and p̄
ctx
   int. monitoring standard:
palpate ctx and
auscultate FHT ✗
  Q 15-30min

Helga (Cont.):
After Shower

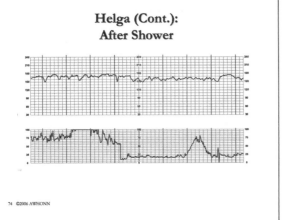

74 ©2006 AWHONN

maternal pain and/or
anxiety can cause fetal
tachycardia d/t
release of catecholemines

Helga (Cont.):
After Fentanyl

75 ©2006 AWHONN

Latoya, 17 years old
G1, P0, 38 weeks gestation

- History: Unremarkable
- Family History: Unremarkable
- Current Status:
  - SROM 1 hour prior to admission, occasional contractions

76 ©2006 AWHONN

clear fluid
fem + nit + VSS afeb

Latoya (Cont.)

Current Pregnancy
- Prenatal course uncomplicated
- 12 prenatal visits
- Two ultrasounds confirmed date and size

12-15 visits isnl. for uncomp preg.

77 ©2006 AWHONN

Latoya (Cont.):
Admission Tracing

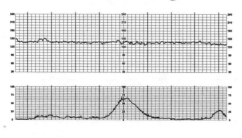

78 ©2006 AWHONN

135 mod. var.
Ø decels
bcc. ctx

2cm
130 mod + accels
∅ decels ireg ctx

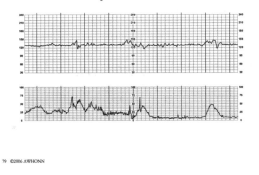

Latoya (Cont.):
Oxytocin Started

140 min. variability
early decels
variable decels

WTF?

∅

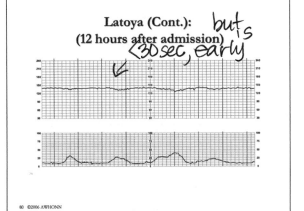

Latoya (Cont.):
(12 hours after admission)
but's
<30 sec, early

Mechanism of Early Deceleration

Pressure on the fetal head
↓
↑ Intracranial pressure
↓
Alteration in cerebral blood flow
↓
Central vagal stimulation
↓
FHR deceleration

Adapted from *Fetal Heart Rate Monitoring* (2nd ed), (p. 13), by R. K. Freeman, T. J. Garite, and M. P. Nageotte, 1991, Baltimore: Williams & Wilkins, reprinted with permission.

Latoya (Cont.)

82 ©2006 AWHONN

Mary, 30 years old
G1, P0, 38 weeks gestation

- History: Unremarkable

- Current Pregnancy: Prenatal period unremarkable

- In Hospital

  > Spontaneous rupture of membranes
    2 hours prior to admission

  > 98° F (36.7° C) temperature, other vital signs
    within normal limits

83 ©2006 AWHONN

Mary: Admission Tracing

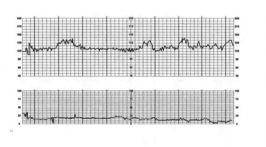

84 ©2006 AWHONN

Max 5 ctx in 10 min is adeq.

hyperstim: persistant pattern
> 5/10
ctx 2 min or more
  ctx within 1 min of each other
may or may not include NRFHR

Mary (Cont.): EFM Reapplied

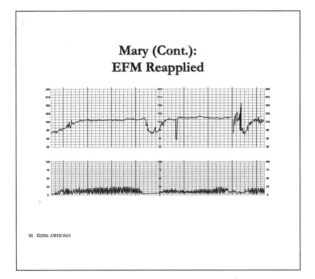

85 ©2006 AWHONN

Mary (Cont.): Toco Readjusted

86 ©2006 AWHONN

Mechanism of Variable Deceleration

PO = Partial Obstruction

CO = Complete Obstruction

UV = Umbilical Vein

UA = Umbilical Artery

FSBP = Fetal Systemic Blood Pressure

(Reprinted with permission from the American College of Obstetricians and Gynecologists [*Obstetrics and Gynecology*, 1975, 45(2), p. 145]).

87 ©2006 AWHONN

variables assoc c̄ ∗ cord compression + ↓ cord perfusion

UV compressed first 2° thin wall, causes fetal BP to ↓.

Mechanism of Variable Deceleration

PO = Partial Obstruction
CO = Complete Obstruction
UV = Umbilical Vein
UA = Umbilical Artery
FSBP = Fetal Systemic Blood Pressure

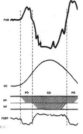

(Reprinted with permission from the American College of Obstetricians and Gynecologists [*Obstetrics and Gynecology*, 1975, 45(2), p. 145]).

88 ©2006 AWHONN

vagus nerve triggered

Mechanism of Variable Deceleration

PO = Partial Obstruction
CO = Complete Obstruction
UV = Umbilical Vein
UA = Umbilical Artery
FSBP = Fetal Systemic Blood Pressure

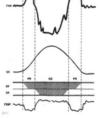

(Reprinted with permission from the American College of Obstetricians and Gynecologists [*Obstetrics and Gynecology*, 1975, 45(2), p. 145])

89 ©2006 AWHONN

ctx subsides
baroreceptors
chemoreceptors
SNS ↑ HR

Mary (Cont.):
Tracing of Variable Shapes

90 ©2006 AWHONN

Fetal Pulse Oximetry Tracing

FSpO2 44%   FSpO2 41%   FSpO2 44%   FSpO2 44%

91 ©2006 AWHONN

PO₂ line — should be ↑30

**Mary (Cont.):
Pushing**

92 ©2006 AWHONN

Non-reassuring requires expedited delivery

mod variability strongly predictive of non-acidemic vigorous infant — even c̄ decels
decreased variability is indicative of acidemia esp. in setting of rep. decels

**Rita, 26 years old
G1 P0, 40 2/7 weeks gestation**

Family History

- Maternal grandmother: Hypertension
- Maternal grandfather: Cardiac disease
- Father of baby in good health

93 ©2006 AWHONN

Rita (Cont.)

- Medical History
  - Exercise-induced asthma
  - Spastic colon
- Current pregnancy
  - Routine prenatal care
  - Prenatal labs: Normal values

94 ©2006 AWHONN

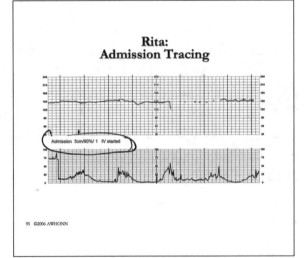

Rita: Admission Tracing

Admission 5cm/90%/ 1 IV started

95 ©2006 AWHONN

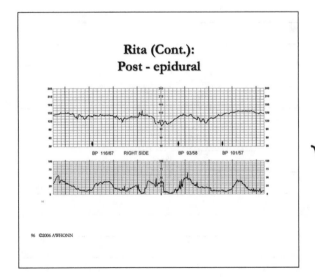

Rita (Cont.): Post - epidural

BP 116/87   RIGHT SIDE   BP 93/58   BP 101/57

96 ©2006 AWHONN

lates
visually apparent
gradual decel
$\geq$ 30 sec

result of
↓ uteroplacental flow

hypotension
pain/anxiety
excessive uterine activity

Rita (Cont.)

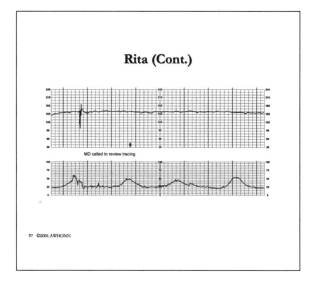

97 ©2006 AWHONN

apgars 2,6,7

Mechanism of Late Decelerations

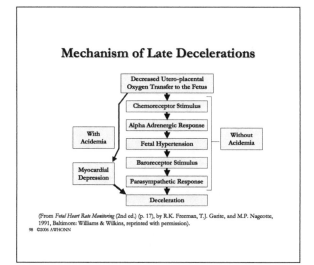

(From *Fetal Heart Rate Monitoring* (2nd ed.) (p. 17), by R.K. Freeman, T.J. Garite, and M.P. Nageotte, 1991, Baltimore: Williams & Wilkins, reprinted with permission).
98 ©2006 AWHONN

in normoxic fetus late decels following an acute insult will usually resolve c̄ tx

recurrent intermittent ↓ in utero-placental flow ↓ reserve

Supine Hypotension

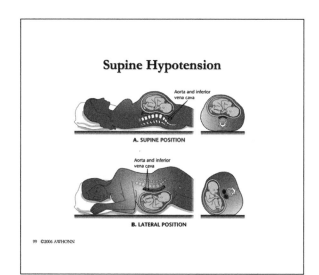

99 ©2006 AWHONN

LL or RL are equally ok

Jane, 40 years old
G3 P2002, 42 weeks gestation

- History
  - Poor nutritional status
  - 2 living children, delivered at 40 and 41 weeks, respectively
- Current Pregnancy
  - 3 prenatal visits
  - Smokes ½ pack of cigarettes per day
  - Poor nutritional status
  - 8 lbs. (3.6 kg) weight gain

100 ©2006 AWHONN

Jane (Cont.)

Current Pregnancy

- Vaginal exam: 2cm/80%/-1
- Premature rupture of membranes >12 hours, clear fluid, no odor
- 98.4° F (36.9° C) temperature

101 ©2006 AWHONN

Jane:
Admission Tracing

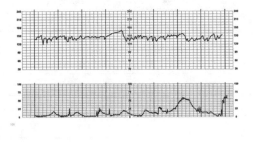

102 ©2006 AWHONN

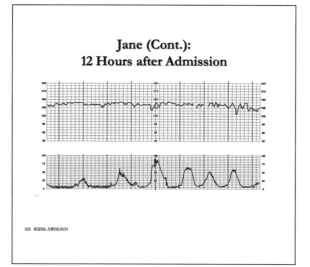

Jane (Cont.):
12 Hours after Admission

103 ©2006 AWHONN

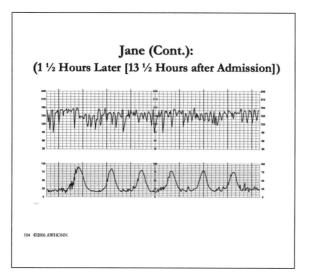

Jane (Cont.):
(1 ½ Hours Later [13 ½ Hours after Admission])

104 ©2006 AWHONN

marked variability
indicative of
fetal sympathetic
stimulation

compensating for
hypoxemia
fetal pO2 ↓ing
uterine hyperstim ↓
placental flow

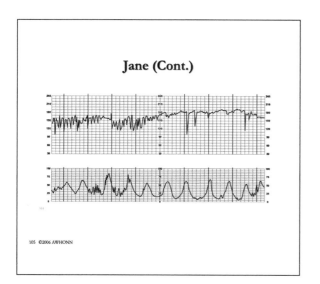

Jane (Cont.)

105 ©2006 AWHONN

**Oxytocin Administration
Based on the Cumulative
Body of Physiologic
and Pharmacologic
Evidence**

106 ©2006 AWHONN

Endogenous Oxytocin

- First stage of labor
  - Maternal circulating concentrations approximately = 2 to 4 mU/min
- Fetal contribution
  - Secretion similar to 3 mU/min
- Combined effects = 5 to 7 mU/min
- Second stage of labor
  - Surge of oxytocin at Ferguson's reflex

107 ©2006 AWHONN

Response to Exogenous Oxytocin

- Initial incremental phase (1.5 to 2 hrs)
  - Uterine contractions will progressively increase in frequency and intensity.
- Stable phase (3.5 to 4.5 hrs)
  - Any further increase will not cause more frequent normal changes in uterine activity but may result in side effects (hyperstimulation/nonreassuring FHR).

108 ©2006 AWHONN

Simpson art
ACOG practice bulletin
2007 study myometrial
receptors

Response to Exogenous Oxytocin

- Oxytocin receptor sites decrease significantly during prolonged oxytocin-induced or augmented labor compared to spontaneous labor.
- Desensitization is related to dosage rate and length of administration.
- More oxytocin for dysfunctional labor will cause further desensitization.
- A rest period of 1 - 2 hours is recommended.

(Phaneuf et al., 2000)

109 ©2006 AWHONN

Pharmacokinetics

- Half-life 10 to 12 minutes
- 3 to 4 half-lives are needed to reach steady-state plasma concentration
- Full effect of oxytocin cannot be evaluated until steady-state concentration has been achieved
- Basis for recommendations for 30 to 40 minute interval dosing of oxytocin

110 ©2006 AWHONN

Oxytocin Dosage

Based on the evidence:

- Physiologic dose is best
  - ➤ 90% of women will achieve active labor at less than 6 mU/min.
  - ➤ Most women do not need more than 10 mU/min.
- At least 30 to 40 minutes between increases is optimal
- No data that more oxytocin will improve dysfunctional labor

Crane & Young (1998); Daniel-Speigel (2004); Phaneuf (2000); Simpson (2002)

111 ©2006 AWHONN

Oxytocin Dosage

Based on the evidence:

- Continuing oxytocin after active labor is established will not shorten labor.

- Long duration and high dose may have opposite intended effect on the course of labor by desensitizing uterine receptors to exogenous & endogenous oxytocin.

- Labor is generally self-sustaining once the active phase is established.

112 ©2006 AWHONN

Evidence-Based Protocol

- Start at 1mU/min

- Increase by 1 - 2 mU/min. q 30 to 40 mins.

- Contractions q 2 to 3 mins.

- Labor progress

- Active Labor: decrease dose or discontinue

- Titrate to fetal and uterine response

- Avoid hyperstimulation; treat before nonreassuring FHR develops whenever possible

113 ©2006 AWHONN

Tina, 26 years old
G1 P0, 39 weeks gestation

- History: Unremarkable

114 ©2006 AWHONN

Tina (Cont.)

Current Pregnancy

- 15 prenatal visits
- 30 lbs. (13.6 kg) weight gain
- SROM at 0650, clear fluid, no odor
- Vaginal exam: 5cm/100%/0
- Vital signs WNL: T 98° F (36.7° C)

115 ©2006 AWHONN

Tina:
Admission Tracing (0719)

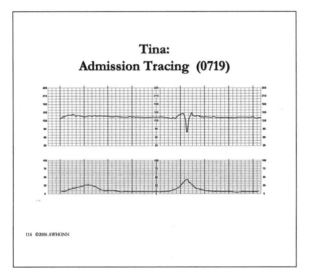

116 ©2006 AWHONN

Tina (Cont.): 0835
(Vaginal exam: 8cm/100%/+1)

117 ©2006 AWHONN

Tina (Cont.): 0850

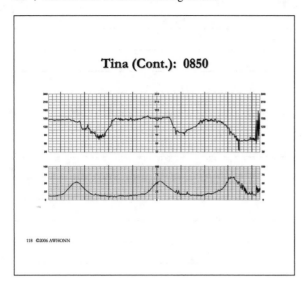

118 ©2006 AWHONN

The Nursing Process and Fetal Monitoring

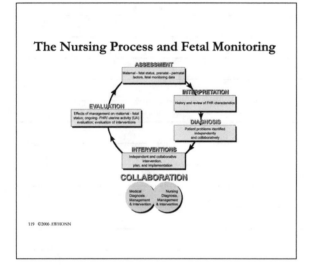

119 ©2006 AWHONN

AWHONN
Association of Women's Health,
Obstetric and Neonatal Nurses

Techniques of
Fetal Heart Monitoring

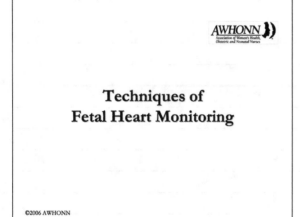

©2006 AWHONN

Margaret, 23 years old
G1 P0, 40 1/7 weeks gestation

- History: Unremarkable
- Current Pregnancy
  - ➢ + Group B Strep by urine culture
    at 36 weeks gestation
  - ➢ 61 lbs. (27.7 kg) pregnancy weight gain

121 ©2006 AWHONN

Margaret: Labor Admission

- Admission for oxytocin induction
- Vital signs: BP 110/62, P 94, T 97.5° F (36.4° C)
- Vaginal exam: 4 cm/90%/-1 station
- Membranes intact
- Method of monitoring
  - ➢ Auscultation and palpation until physician arrival

122 ©2006 AWHONN

Benefits of Auscultation

- Detects FHR baseline rate and rhythm, as well as
  increases and decreases of the FHR
- Widespread application
- Compares favorably with EFM
- Not subject to machine error
- Noninvasive
- Allows patient freedom of movement and ambulation

123 ©2006 AWHONN

Benefits of Auscultation (Cont.)

- Increased hands-on time with patient
- Verification of FHR dysrhythmias visualized on EFM tracing (fetoscope)
- Clarification of halving or doubling on the EFM tracing
- Differentiates fetal and maternal heart rates, eliminating errors due to misplaced monitoring devices or fetal demise

124 ©2006 AWHONN

Limitations of Auscultation

- Auscultation not continuous and may miss or delay detection of FHR increases & decreases
- Does not detect fetal heart rate variability
- FHR assessment may be limited by position or movement of mother and fetus; and maternal size
- Uterine tension disrupts assessment
- Requires education, practice, skill, 1:1 nurse/patient ratio
- No copy generated for collaborative decision making and record keeping

125 ©2006 AWHONN

Margaret (Cont.)

Auscultation Findings

- Rate: 130s - 140s
- Rhythm: Regular
- Increases in FHR to 150s - 170s
- No decreases auscultated

Palpation Findings

- No palpable contractions
- Resting tone soft

126 ©2006 AWHONN

Margaret (Cont.)

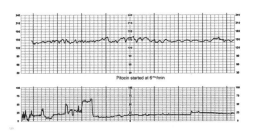

Pitocin started at 6 mu/min

127 ©2006 AWHONN

Benefits of Ultrasound Transducer

- Noninvasive, no need to rupture membranes
- Relatively consistent recordings if placed correctly
- FHR recorded for future comparison and permanent record
- Less personnel-intensive than auscultation: Is this a plus or a minus?

128 ©2006 AWHONN

Limitations of the Ultrasound Transducer

- Less personnel intensive; may decrease provider time at the bedside
- Restricts patient movement
- Maternal/fetal movement may interfere with recording.
- Limited by maternal size or position
- Ultrasound reflections may be weak or absent
- Maternal heart rate may be recorded erroneously.
- FHR may half or double count when profound tachycardia and bradycardia are present.

129 ©2006 AWHONN

Machine Half and Double Counting

- Greater than 240 bpm
- Less than 30 bpm
- Maternal or fetal heart rate may be halved or doubled under certain conditions.

130 ©2006 AWHONN

Example of Machine Error
Half Counting

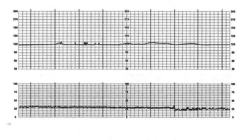

131 ©2006 AWHONN

Margaret (Cont.)

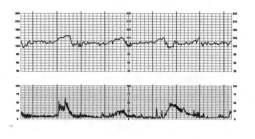

132 ©2006 AWHONN

Margaret (Cont.)

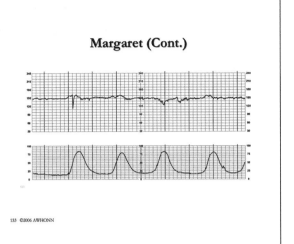

133 ©2006 AWHONN

Benefits of Spiral Electrode

- Continuous detection of FHR
- Detection of dysrhythmias more likely
- Maternal position changes do not affect tracing quality.

134 ©2006 AWHONN

Limitations of Spiral Electrode

- Necessitates rupture of membranes, cervical dilatation and an accessible/acceptable presenting part
- Electronic interference and artifact may occur
- Small risk of fetal hemorrhage or infection
- May be contraindicated in certain maternal-fetal conditions

135 ©2006 AWHONN

Limitations of Spiral Electrode (Cont.)

- Requires moist environment for detection of fetal heart rate
- May record maternal HR in presence of fetal demise
- May miss fetal dysrhythmias if logic or ECG button engaged

136 ©2006 AWHONN

Margaret (Cont.)

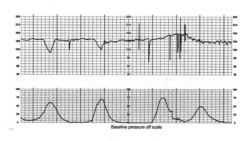

Baseline pressure off scale

137 ©2006 AWHONN

Margaret: Outcome

- Cesarean birth
- Male infant
- Birth weight: 9 lbs., 11 oz. (4,394 gm)
- Apgar scores of 8 and 9

138 ©2006 AWHONN

Pat, 32 years old
G6 P3204, weeks gestation unclear

- History
  - Chronic hypertension
  - Previous twins died in infancy
- Current Pregnancy
  - No prenatal care
  - Suspected intrauterine growth restriction (IUGR)
  - Vital signs: 134/92, 80, 97.5 °F (36.4 °C)
  - Albumin negative

139 ©2006 AWHONN

Pat:
Admission Tracing

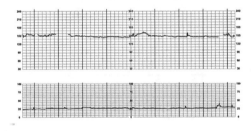

140 ©2006 AWHONN

Definition of Palpation

**Assessment of uterine contractions
by discriminating the change in intensity
of the contraction of the uterus**

141 ©2006 AWHONN

Comparison Model for Palpation of Uterine Activity

Palpation of Uterus	Feels Like	Contraction Intensity
Easily indented	Tip of nose	Mild
Can slightly indent	Chin	Moderate
Cannot indent	Forehead	Strong

142 ©2006 AWHONN

Benefits of Palpation

- Measures contraction frequency, duration and relative strength
- Widely used
- Provides hands-on assessment and care of the patient
- Allows patient freedom of movement and ambulation
- Noninvasive

143 ©2006 AWHONN

Pat (Cont.)

Plan of care
- Continuous fetal monitoring
- Daily fetal movement count
- Biophysical profile

144 ©2006 AWHONN

Pat (Cont.)

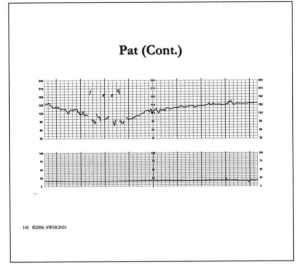

145 ©2006 AWHONN

Pat (Cont.)

Plan of Care

- Amniocentesis results: Immature lungs
- Steroid dosing
- Continuous fetal monitoring

146 ©2006 AWHONN

Pat (Cont.): Day 5

- Amniocentesis mature
- Diastolic BP range: 100 -105 mmHg
- Vaginal exam: 2-3 cm/50%/-1
- Continued prolonged decelerations
- Plan: Oxytocin induction

147 ©2006 AWHONN

Benefits of Tocodynamometry

- Noninvasive and easily placed
- Does not require ruptured membranes
- Records relative measurement of contraction frequency & duration when placed correctly
- Uterine activity recorded for future review and permanent record

148 ©2006 AWHONN

Limitations of Tocodynamometry

- Location-sensitive; placement can lead to false information
- Data limited to frequency and duration but not intensity or resting tone
- Maternal/fetal movement may interfere with data
- Limits patient's freedom to move
- Gestational age and maternal size may limit data obtained

149 ©2006 AWHONN

Limitations of Palpation

- Subjective
- Requires practice to achieve proficiency
- No copy generated for collaborative decision making and record keeping
- Maternal movement and intolerance may interfere and assessment
- Limited by maternal size

150 ©2006 AWHONN

Benefits of Intrauterine Pressure Catheter (IUPC)

- Accurate assessment of frequency, duration, intensity of contractions, and of resting tone
- Withdrawal of amniotic fluid for testing
- Amnioinfusion port
- May be recalibrated or flushed to validate accuracy of internal monitoring

151 ©2006 AWHONN

Limitations of Intrauterine Pressure Catheter (IUPC)

- Invasive procedure
- Need ruptured membranes, cervical dilatation
- Increased risk of infection and/or uterine perforation
- Placement of IUPC and maternal position affect baseline and contraction pressures

152 ©2006 AWHONN

Limitations of IUPC (Cont.)

- Difference in readings between fluid-filled and sensor-tipped catheters
- Catheter can become obstructed or wedged, preventing the pressure wave reading
- Contraindicated with some presentations, stations, significant bleeding or infection

153 ©2006 AWHONN

Pat (Cont.)

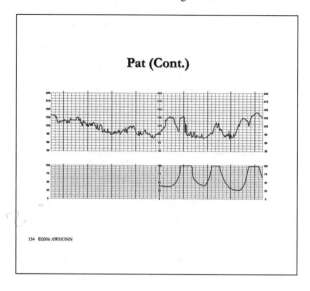

154 ©2006 AWHONN

Pat (Cont.)

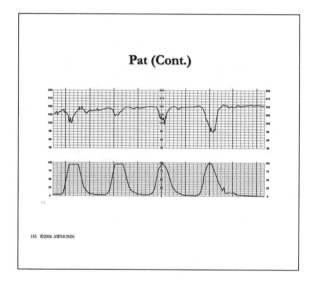

155 ©2006 AWHONN

Pat: Outcome

- Cesarean birth
- Male infant
- Apgar scores of 8 and 9
- Birth weight: 3.04 lbs. (1,380 gm)
- IUGR
- 10% abruption

156 ©2006 AWHONN

Troubleshooting

- Is this machine artifact?
- Is this a FHR dysrhythmia?
- Is this a nonreassuring pattern?

157 ©2006 AWHONN

Nicole, 27 years old
G1 P0, 39 weeks gestation

- History: Unremarkable
- Current Pregnancy
  - Serial ultrasounds at 18, 30, 34 and 36 weeks asymmetrical IUGR
  - Vaginal exam: 3 cm/90%/0

158 ©2006 AWHONN

Nicole:
Admission Tracing

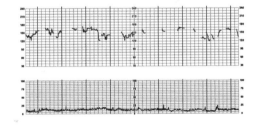

159 ©2006 AWHONN

Unable to assess tracing due to poor quality

Troubleshooting the Ultrasound

- Confirm fetal position by Leopold's maneuvers
- Auscultate the FHR
- Reapply monitor gel
- Reposition the transducer to detect fetal cardiac motion
- Reposition the mother
- Real-time ultrasound visualization
- Apply fetal spiral electrode (FSE)

160 ©2006 AWHONN

Troubleshooting the Tocodynamometer

- Palpate for the point of strongest fundal intensity.
- Place the toco flat and firm against the abdomen.
- Check monitor equipment.
- Consider intrauterine pressure catheter monitoring.

161 ©2006 AWHONN

Nicole (Cont.)

162 ©2006 AWHONN

Nicole (Cont.)

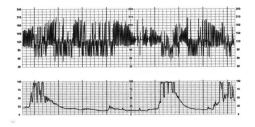

Troubleshooting the Spiral Electrode

- Listen to what your ears are telling you.
- Check connections to the monitor, electrode cable, presenting part.
- Check the circuitry.
- Check the on/off position of logic or electrocardiogram (ECG) disable switch.
- Confirm the maternal pulse.
- Auscultate with fetoscope to confirm the FHR.
- Change the FSE.

Nicole (Cont.): SE, IUPC

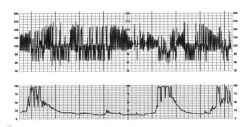

Troubleshooting the IUPC

- Verify IUPC position (check markings at perineum and ask patient to cough)
- Flush catheter (if applicable)
- Recalibrate if:
  - Resting tone too high/too low despite palpation of soft uterus
  - No contraction pattern with palpable contractions
  - Artifact present
- Check monitor for loose connections or re-zero IUPC prn
- Run monitor's self-test feature

166 ©2006 AWHONN

Documentation

- Initial FHR tracing
- Troubleshooting steps
- Current fetal status and uterine contraction pattern

167 ©2006 AWHONN

Nicole: Outcome

- Spontaneous vaginal birth
- Female infant
- Apgar scores of 8 and 9
- 5 lbs., 7 oz. (2,466 gm)
- Cord blood pH 7.23, 7.26, arterial and venous, respectively
- Normal heart rhythm at 1 hour of age
- Home with mother

168 ©2006 AWHONN

Care and Storage of Equipment

- Handle with caution due to fragile nature.
- Never immerse transducers or cables in water, unless indicated by manufacturer.
- Clean monitor, transducers, and cables with approved disinfectant.
- Loosely coil cables for storage.
- Don't force insertion of cables into monitor if they don't fit.
- Dispose or wash fetal monitor straps according to facility or manufacturers' recommendations.

169 ©2006 AWHONN

Techniques Summary

- Methods for assessing FHR
- Methods for assessing uterine contractions
- Troubleshooting monitor information

170 ©2006 AWHONN

AWHONN
Association of Women's Health,
Obstetric and Neonatal Nurses

Choosing Physiologically Based Interventions

©2006 AWHONN

Physiologic Goals

- Support maternal coping and labor progress.
- Maximize uterine blood flow.
- Maximize umbilical circulation.
- Maximize oxygenation.
- Maintain appropriate uterine activity.

172 ©2006 AWHONN

Interventions to Support Coping and Labor Progress

- Review plans/expectations with the woman and her partner, friends, or family.
- Maintain calm environment whenever possible
- Include family members where appropriate.
- Stay at the bedside as much as possible.
- Monitor only at the level needed for this patient.
- Use frequent position changes, upright positioning.
- Minimize use of technology; avoid unnecessary intervention.

173 ©2006 AWHONN

Interventions to Maximize Uterine Blood Flow

- Anxiety/pain reduction
- Maternal position change
- Hydration
- Medication

174 ©2006 AWHONN

Interventions to Maximize Umbilical Circulation

- Maternal position change
- Elevation of presenting part
- Amnioinfusion

175 ©2006 AWHONN

Interventions to Maximize Oxygenation

- Maternal position change
- Maternal supplemental oxygen
- Maternal hydration
- Maternal breathing techniques
- Correct or treat underlying disease

176 ©2006 AWHONN

Maternal–Fetal Response to Pain

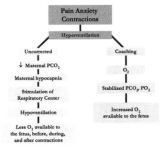

177 ©2006 AWHONN

Interventions to
Modify Uterine Activity

- Maternal position change
- Appropriate use of uterotonic drugs
- Hydration
- Tocolytic medication
- Appropriate second stage of labor care

178 ©2006 AWHONN

Physiology of the Second Stage of Labor

```
Long          ↑Abdominal      ↑Vasoconstriction    Maternal
Valsalva      and                                   Blood      ──→   Blood Flow
Maneuver  ──→ Intrathoracic ──→ ↓Cardiac Output  ── Flow ──→         in the
              Pressure                                                Intervillous
                              ↑Intrauterine        Uterine           Space
                              Pressure          ── Blood
                                                   Flow

Blood Flow in the        ↓pH, pO₂          ↑Newborn
Intervillous        ──→  Base Excess  ──→  Acidemia
Space                    ↑pCO₂             ↓Apgar
                         Nonreassuring     Scores
                         FHR
```

(Adapted from Barnett, M.M. & Humenick S.S. (1982). Infant outcome in relation to second stage labor pushing method. *Birth.* 9: 221-229.).
179 ©2006 AWHONN

Changes in FSpO2 with Pushing

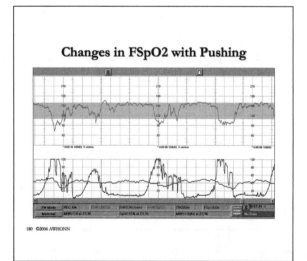

180 ©2006 AWHONN

The Second Stage of Labor

- Two phases
  - Initial latent phase
  - Active pushing phase
- Wait until urge to push before assisting with pushing efforts.
- Take advantage of latent phase to let the fetus descend and the mother rest.

181 ©2006 AWHONN

Support Rather than Direct

- Support involuntary pushing:
  - Delay pushing and defer coaching whenever possible.
- If need for direction is demonstrated:
  - Discourage prolonged breath holding.
  - Discourage more than 3 pushing efforts.
  - Limit pushing efforts to 6 - 8 seconds each.
  - Don't discourage grunting and vocalization.

182 ©2006 AWHONN

Supporting the Fetus in the Active Phase of the Second Stage

- Take steps to maintain a reassuring FHR pattern while pushing
- Push with every other or every third contraction if necessary to help avoid recurrent FHR decelerations
- Reposition frequently to promote progress
- Use the usual intrauterine resuscitation techniques when needed
- Avoid uterine hyperstimulation
- Avoid valsalva pushing

183 ©2006 AWHONN

Betty, 33 years old
G2 P1001, 39 weeks gestation

- Presented with vaginal bleeding.
- Complained of decreased fetal movement.
- Ultrasound done. Placenta previa ruled out.
- Vaginal exam: 3 cm/80%/-2, and vertex presentation
- AROM. Large amount thin green fluid
- SE and IUPC applied.

184 ©2006 AWHONN

Betty (Cont.):
Tracing at 1 Hour Post Admission

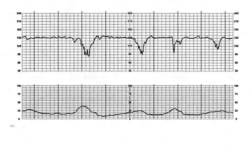

185 ©2006 AWHONN

Betty (Cont.)

Physiologic Goal

Maximize umbilical circulation.

186 ©2006 AWHONN

Interventions

- Change maternal position.
- Palpate contractions and verify the IUPC.
- Perform vaginal exam as indicated.
- Recheck maternal vital signs.
- Inform/support woman and her family.
- Confer with Betty's other providers (CNM/MD).

187 ©2006 AWHONN

True Knot in Cord

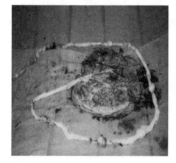

188 ©2006 AWHONN

Cord Entanglement

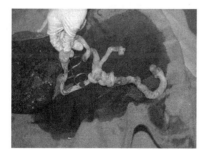

189 ©2006 AWHONN

Amnioinfusion

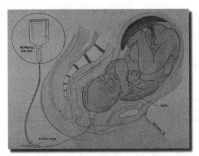

190 ©2006 AWHONN

Marsha, 20 years old
G2 P1001, 39 weeks gestation

- History: Unremarkable
- Current pregnancy
  - No risk factors
  - Admitted in early labor
  - Vaginal exam: 2 cm/80%/-1; spontaneous rupture of membranes, clear fluid, no odor
  - Uterine contractions every 3 min. x 60 - 70 sec, moderate by palpation

191 ©2006 AWHONN

Marsha (Cont.)

- Regional anesthesia at 11:45 (sitting position)
- Vital signs: 100/58, 98, 98.6° F (37° C)

192 ©2006 AWHONN

Marsha (Cont.):
15 Minutes Later

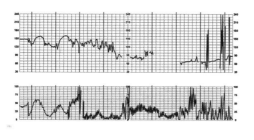

193 ©2006 AWHONN

Bradycardia:
Immediate Interventions

- Call for help and notify primary care provider.
- Perform vaginal exam.
- Prepare to expedite birth.
- Initiate intrauterine resuscitation:
  - ➢ Change maternal position and palpate uterus
  - ➢ Oxygenate
  - ➢ Hydrate
  - ➢ Assess BP: Medicate as indicated/ordered

194 ©2006 AWHONN

Mechanism of Intrauterine Resuscitation with Terbutaline

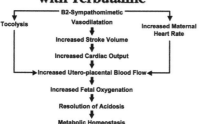

(From Intrauterine resuscitation of the fetus by A. P. Sarno & J. P. Phelan, 1988. *Contemporary OB/GYN, 31*(7), 143-152. Reprinted with permission.)

195 ©2006 AWHONN

Marsha (Cont.)

Significant Physiology

- Hypotension?
- Compression of umbilical cord?
- Excessive uterine activity?
- Abruption?
- Sudden descent?

196 ©2006 AWHONN

Marsha (Cont.)

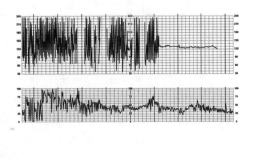

197 ©2006 AWHONN

Fetal Scalp Stimulation Example

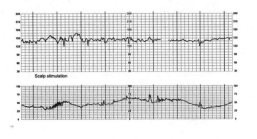

Scalp stimulation

198 ©2006 AWHONN

Vera, 32 years old
G4 P2012, 36 weeks gestation

- History: Unremarkable
- Current pregnancy
  - Chicken pox at 6-8 weeks gestation
  - Ultrasound at 32 and 35 weeks gestation with body in < 10th, and BPD in 28th percentile
  - Current pregnancy history otherwise unremarkable
  - Admitted for labor induction IUGR

199 ©2006 AWHONN

Vera (Cont.)

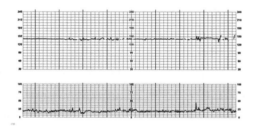

200 ©2006 AWHONN

Interventions:
Minimal Variability on Admission

- Change maternal position.
- Oxygenate.
- Hydrate.
- Ask about change in fetal movement.
- Call for bedside evaluation.

201 ©2006 AWHONN

Placental and Umbilical Blood Vessel Gas Exchange

Uterine artery
PO$_2$ 100 mm Hg
PCO$_2$ 32 mm Hg
pH 7.42

Umbilical arteries
PO$_2$ 17 mm Hg
PCO$_2$ 53 mm Hg
pH 7.26

Uterine vein
PO$_2$ 40 mm Hg
PCO$_2$ 46 mm Hg
pH 7.30

Umbilical vein
PO$_2$ 29 mm Hg
PCO$_2$ 41 mm Hg
pH 7.34

202 ©2006 AWHONN

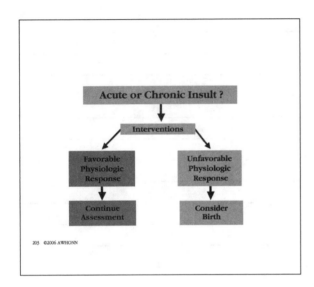

Acute or Chronic Insult ?

Interventions

Favorable Physiologic Response

Unfavorable Physiologic Response

Continue Assessment

Consider Birth

203 ©2006 AWHONN

Vera (Cont.)

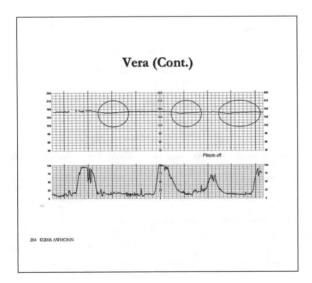

Pitocin off

204 ©2006 AWHONN

Vera: Outcome

- Emergent cesarean birth
- Infant boy weighing 4 lbs., 9 oz (2,070 gm)
- Baby initially vigorous, Apgar scores of 8 and 9
- Infant assessment at birth revealed multiple chicken pox scars on trunk and extremities.
- Transferred to a tertiary care center
- Neurologic deficit diagnosed after transfer.

205 ©2006 AWHONN

Vera (Cont.)

Arterial Cord Blood Gas Results

- pH   7.32
- pCO_2 44.1
- pO_2 20.2
- Bicarbonate   22.0
- Base deficit (BD) 3.7

206 ©2006 AWHONN

Chou Le, 28 years old
G3 P1011, 36 weeks gestation

History

- 1 miscarriage at 6 weeks
- 1 spontaneous vaginal birth at 39 weeks, child now 6 years old
- Type 1 diabetes
  - Family history of Type I diabetes
  - Mother has Type 1 diabetes

207 ©2006 AWHONN

Chou Le (Cont.)

Current Pregnancy

- 15 prenatal visits
- On NPH and regular insulin
- Blood sugars well managed
- 35 lbs. (15.9 kg) pregnancy weight gain
- 4 days ago: Reactive nonstress test
- Biophysical profile today: 2/10
- Grade III placenta

208 ©2006 AWHONN

Chou Le:
Admission Tracing

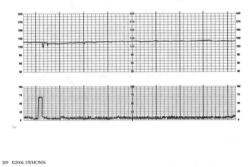

209 ©2006 AWHONN

Chou Le (Cont.):
Tracing 45 Minutes Later

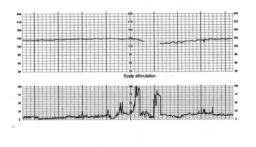

210 ©2006 AWHONN

Chou Le (Cont.)

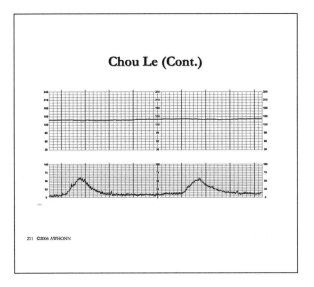

211 ©2006 AWHONN

Chou Le (Cont.)
Final tracing

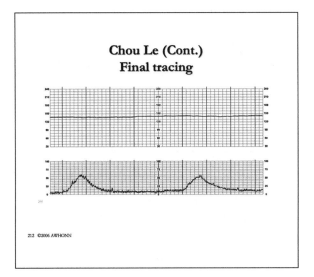

212 ©2006 AWHONN

Single-Digit Value Guideline
Initial Assessment of Umbilical Cord Blood Acid-Base Values

	Target Values	Metabolic Acidemia	Respiratory Acidemia
pH	≥ 7.10	< 7.10	< 7.10
pO2 (mmHg)	> 20	< 20	variable
pCO2 (mmHg)	< 60	< 60	> 60
Bicarbonate (mEq/L)	> 22	< 22	≥ 22
BD (mEq/L)	≤ 12	> 12	< 12
BE (mEq/L)	≥ -12	< -12	> -12

213 ©2006 AWHONN

Types of Acidosis

	pH	pCO2	pO2	BD
Respiratory	↓	↑	Variable	WNL
Metabolic	↓	WNL	↓	↑
Mixed	↓	↑	↓	↑

214 ©2006 AWHONN

Chou Le

Arterial Cord Blood Gas Values

- Apgar scores   1 and 5
- pH   7.09
- pO2   15 mmHg
- pCO2   75 mmHg
- BD   12 mEq/L
- Bicarbonate   18 mEq/L

215 ©2006 AWHONN

Elizabeth, 36 years old
G2 P0010, 41 weeks gestation

History

- Spontaneous abortion at 10 weeks gestation

- Current pregnancy

- Admitted with spontaneous rupture of membranes x 12 hours, clear fluid, no odor

- Occasional uterine contractions, mild by palpation

216 ©2006 AWHONN

Elizabeth

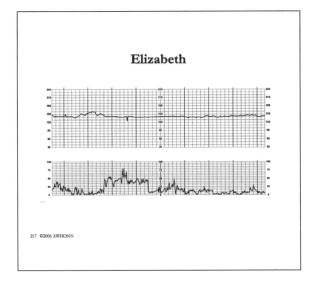

217 ©2006 AWHONN

Elizabeth (Cont.):
3 Hours Later

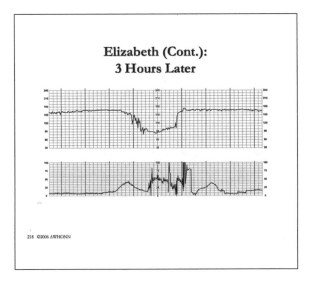

218 ©2006 AWHONN

Elizabeth (Cont.)

Goals

- Reduce uterine activity.
- Maximize oxygenation.
- Maximize uterine blood flow.
- Maximize umbilical circulation.

219 ©2006 AWHONN

Elizabeth (Cont.)

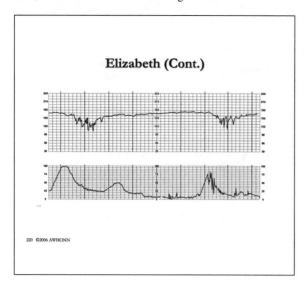

Elizabeth (Cont.)

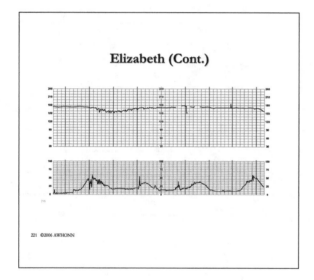

Factors Affecting Fetal Scalp Sampling and Interpretation of Results

- Presentation, position, station
- Dilatation, effacement
- Thick fetal hair
- Financial considerations, equipment, resources

- Time lapse for filling the capillary tube
- Machine calibration
- Maternal acid-base balance requiring comparative fetal samples

Factors Affecting Fetal Scalp Sampling and Interpretation of Results (Cont.)

- Uterine activity at time of sampling
- Fetal trauma due to procedure
- Presence of meconium
- Sampling in area of cephalohematoma, caput or fontanels
- Contamination of sample
- Acceptance and position of mother
- Experience of provider

223 ©2006 AWHONN

Elizabeth: Outcome

Neonatal Arterial Cord Blood Values

pH	7.09
pCO2	80 mmHg
pO2	18 mmHg
BD	15 mEq/L

224 ©2006 AWHONN

Sharice: Admission Tracing

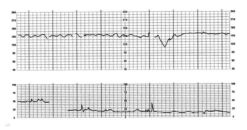

225 ©2006 AWHONN

Karen:
Nonstress test

226 ©2006 AWHONN

Sharice and Karen (Cont.)

Rapid Assessments/Interventions:

- Notify primary care provider and request bedside evaluation.
- Change maternal position.
- Oxygenate.
- Hydrate.
- Palpate uterus.
- Perform further assessment.

227 ©2006 AWHONN

Sharice, 23 years old
G1 P0, 33 weeks gestation

Current Pregnancy

- Complaint of decreased fetal movement
- BPP 2/10:
  - ➤ 2 for amniotic fluid volume
  - ➤ Absent fetal breathing movement (0)
  - ➤ Absent fetal movement (0)
  - ➤ Absent fetal tone (0)
  - ➤ Nonreactive nonstress test (0)

228 ©2006 AWHONN

Sharice (Cont.)

Current Pregnancy

- Cesarean birth
- Baby's Apgar scores of 2, 5, and 7 at 1, 5, and 10 minutes
- Baby very pale with suspected fetal-maternal hemorrhage, unknown source
- Placenta normal: No abruption

229 ©2006 AWHONN

Karen, 26 years old
G4 P3003, 37 weeks gestation

Current Pregnancy

- Complaint of decreased fetal movement
- Ultrasound examination revealed anencephaly

230 ©2006 AWHONN

The Nursing Process and Fetal Monitoring

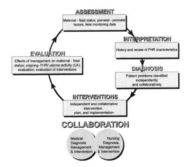

231 ©2006 AWHONN

**Communication and
Accountability**

©2006 AWHONN

Communication

- Is essential and central to quality care
- Primary purpose: meet patient's needs appropriately

233 ©2006 AWHONN

**Essential Principles
of Effective Teamwork**

- In complex environments teams, rather than individuals, create optimal performance.
- Effective teams work collectively to achieve agreed-upon goal: best possible outcome.
- Each team member is valued for their unique experience, knowledge, and contributions.
- Professionals are responsible & accountable for their individual behavior.

234 ©2006 AWHONN

Essential Principles
of Effective Communication

Open   Clear   Honest

Concise   Respectful

Be Direct:

When you know what you need, ask for it!

235 ©2006 AWHONN

Briefings and Assertion

SBAR:

- Situation
- Background
- Assessment
- *Recommendation*

Be Assertive

Get Person's Attention

Express Concern

State Problem

Propose Action

Reach Decision

"I AM CONCERNED"

(Preston P [2004]. Practical perinatal safety: Some high yield interventions. Antepartum & Intrapartum Management Conference, San Francisco, CA, June 19, 2004.)

(Simpson & Knox [2003], *AWHONN Lifelines*)

236 ©2006 AWHONN

Example #1

"Based on my initial assessment, this patient is having variable decelerations and has meconium-stained fluid. May I have an order for an amnioinfusion, and can you please come in to see this patient as soon as possible?"

237 ©2006 AWHONN

Example #2

"I am concerned about your order to start oxytocin because of the nonreassuring fetal heart rate pattern. I am going to wait until you are able to come in and see this patient and we can review the tracing together. When can I expect to see you?"

238 ©2006 AWHONN

Example #3

"I'm calling about Ms. Garcia, the 33 year old woman in labor with preeclampsia we spoke about earlier. Fetal status is deteriorating, and I need you here now."

239 ©2006 AWHONN

Transfers of Care (Hand-offs)

■ Transfers of care are a time of vulnerability
■ Whenever possible:
  ➤ Use face-to-face reporting.
  ➤ Assess patient status together.
  ➤ Solicit oncoming provider's questions, opinion.
  ➤ Provide written summary of critical information:
    ■ Use protocols or checklists to ensure completeness.
    ■ Ensure information is up-to-date & accurate.

240 ©2006 AWHONN

Documentation

- Should be a streamlined, factual and objective record of the care provided.
- Should contain <u>only</u> and <u>all</u> clinically relevant information.
- Duplication of information should be avoided:
  - Whenever possible, avoid documenting routine care on the EFM tracing when it is also being recorded in the chart.
- Detailed description of tracings are unnecessary.

241   ©2006 AWHONN

Documentation (Cont.)

- Should reflect a systematic admission and ongoing assessment of the laboring woman and fetus.
- Assessment and documentation should occur in time frames that are consistent with the patient's condition, as well as institutional and professional guidelines.

242   ©2006 AWHONN

Flow Sheet for FHR Documentation

Date of Record:					
	TIME				
Cervix	Dilation				
	Effacement				
	Station				
Fetal Heart	Baseline Rate				
	Variability				
	Accelerations				
	Decelerations				
	STIM/pH				
	Monitor Mode				
Uterine Activity	Frequency				
	Duration				
	Intensity				
	Resting Tone				
	Monitor Mode				
	Coping				
	Maternal Position				
	O2 L/min/Mask				
	IV				
	Initials				

243   ©2006 AWHONN

Information on EFM Tracing Labels

- Patient name
- Hospital identification number
- Date and time monitoring begun
- Mode of monitoring
- Calibration test, per facility protocol

244 ©2006 AWHONN

Questions About Documenting EFM Assessments

- Frequency of assessment?
- Frequency of documentation?
- Baseline fetal heart rate?
- Variability?
- Periodic FHR changes?
- Contraction pattern?

245 ©2006 AWHONN

Frequency of Electronic Fetal Monitoring Evaluation: LOW-RISK Patients

- This may occur at the same intervals as monitoring with auscultation.
  - ➢ Every 30 minutes during active phase
  - ➢ Every 15 minutes during 2nd stage

(AWHONN, 2000; ACOG, 2005)

246 ©2006 AWHONN

Frequency of Electronic Fetal Monitoring Evaluation - HIGH-RISK patients

- Every 15 minutes during active phase
- Every 5 minutes during the 2nd stage of labor

(AWHONN, 2000; ACOG, 2005)

247 ©2006 AWHONN

Assessment vs. Documentation

KEY POINT:

Assessments are conducted at intervals appropriate to maternal-fetal condition. Documentation does not necessarily have to occur at the same intervals.

248 ©2006 AWHONN

SOGC Guidelines for Fetal Heart Rate Assessment

- Electronic fetal monitoring records should be inspected and documented:
  - ➤ Every 15 minutes during the active phase of labor
  - ➤ At least every 5 minutes during the second stage of labor
- Frequency of auscultation:
  - ➤ Every 15 - 30 minutes in active labor
  - ➤ Every 5 minutes in the active portion of the second stage

(Society of Obstetricians and Gynaecologists of Canada (SOGC), 2002a)

249 ©2006 AWHONN

Suggested Frequency for Auscultation

	Latent Phase	Active Phase	Second Stage
AWHONN		q 15-30 min	q 5 -15 min
ACOG		q 15 min	q 5 min
RCOG		q 15 min	q 5 min
SOGC	Regularly after ROM or other clinically significant change	q 15 -30 min	q 15 min, then q 5 min once pushing initiated

(ACOG, 2005; AWHONN, 2005; Feinstein, Sprague and Trepanier, 2000; RCOG, 2001; SOGC, 2002)

250 ©2006 AWHONN

Fetal Heart Rate Variability

Absent	Undetectable amplitude
Minimal	Visually detectable, but ≤ 5 bpm amplitude
Moderate	6 - 25 bpm amplitude
Marked	> 25 bpm amplitude

251 ©2006 AWHONN

Fetal Heart Rate Baseline

Documented as a single number representing the mean baseline FHR, rounded to the closest 5-beat increment according to the NICHD terminology.

252 ©2006 AWHONN

Baseline 135 bpm, Moderate Variability

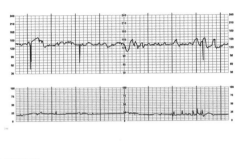

253 ©2006 AWHONN

Baseline 160 bpm, Absent Variability

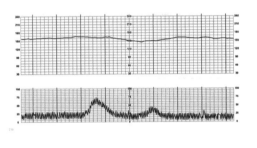

254 ©2006 AWHONN

Documentation of EFM Patterns

- Accelerations
- Early, late and variable decelerations by using their descriptive names
- Recurrence of patterns (repetitiveness)
- Evolution of the pattern over time
- Associated clinical findings

255 ©2006 AWHONN

Clarifying Confusing Patterns

Focus on:

- The baseline variability
- Evolution of the tracing
- Other clinical indicators of fetal well-being and maternal progress in labor
- Maternal-fetal response to interventions

256 ©2006 AWHONN

Documentation of Auscultation

- Numerical rate
- Rhythm
- Decreases or increases in rate
  - Gradual
  - Abrupt
- Timing related to contraction

257 ©2006 AWHONN

Documentation of Uterine Activity

- Uterine Contraction
- Frequency
- Duration
- Intensity
- Resting tonus

258 ©2006 AWHONN

Documentation of Uterine Activity (Cont.)

Toco: Manual Palpation

- Contractions
  - Mild
  - Moderate
  - Strong
- Resting Tone
  - Soft
  - Firm

IUPC

- Actual numbers in mmHg
- Montevideo units (MVU)

259 ©2006 AWHONN

Components of Fetal Monitoring Documentation

- Assessments
- Pertinent events and actions
- Nursing interventions
- Maternal-fetal responses to interventions
- Notification of primary care provider

260 ©2006 AWHONN

Documentation Example

- Repositioned to right side
- IV bolus of 500 ml LR
- O2 at 10 L/min per non-rebreather face mask
- Maternal BP returned to 100/70 from 90/48
- Moderate variability, baseline 155 bpm following interventions
- Dr. _____ notified of above findings.
  Signature

261 ©2006 AWHONN

Critique of Video Segment

Patient Education About
Electronic Fetal Monitoring

262 ©2006 AWHONN

Communication
Patient Teaching about EFM

- Inform mother and partner about purpose and method of electronic monitoring
- Discuss FHR tracing and usual baseline rate
- Discuss uterine contraction tracing and timing of contractions
- Explain volume control
- Explain positioning and implications for ambulation as appropriate

263 ©2006 AWHONN

Dawn, 24 years old
G2 P1001, 38 3/7 weeks gestation

- History: Unremarkable
- Current Pregnancy
  - Twins (dichorionic/diamniotic)
  - No other risk factors

264 ©2006 AWHONN

Dawn: Tracing of twins

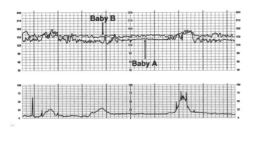

265 ©2006 AWHONN

Dawn: Flow Sheet Documentation of Twins

Date of Record	4/16/2002				
	TIME		1:00		
		:15			
Cervix	Dilation				
	Effacement				
	Station				
Fetal Heart	Baseline Rate	A 144 / B 155			
	Variability	A Mod / B Mod			
	Accelerations	+/+			
	Decelerations	none			
	STIM/pH				
	Monitor Mode				
Uterine Activity	Frequency	q 3-5			
	Duration	50-80 sec			
	Intensity	25-60 mmHg			
	Resting Tone	5-15 mmHg			
	Monitor Mode	EUPC			
	Coping	Well			
	Maternal Position	Sitting			
	O2 L/min/Mask				
	IV				
	Initials	NN			

266 ©2006 AWHONN

Dawn: Alternative Documentation

Baby A:
BL 140 bpm; moderate variability; + accels

Baby B:
BL 155 bpm; moderate variability; + accels

Uterine contractions every 3 - 5 min. x 50 - 80 sec., 25 - 60 mmHg, resting tone 5 - 15 mmHg

F.S.W., RN

267 ©2006 AWHONN

Beth, 29 years old
G3 P1101, 38 weeks gestation

- History
  - Previous preterm birth at 23 weeks, nonviable
  - Previous term birth at 39 weeks, living and well
- Current Pregnancy
  - No risk factors other than history of preterm labor
  - Reason for admission: SROM, scant green fluid

268 ©2006 AWHONN

Beth (Cont.)

- Vital signs: 126/68, 78, 18, 98.2° F (36.7° C)
- Uterine contractions every 4 - 5 min. x 40-50 sec; mild-moderate by palpation
- Vaginal exam: 4 cm/80%/-1, vertex
- US & toco applied
- Comfortable

269 ©2006 AWHONN

Beth: Admission Tracing

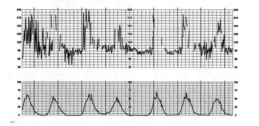

270 ©2006 AWHONN

Communication Nurse and Beth

- How will you talk with her?
- How will you answer questions?
- What questions can you ask to get more information?
- What will you document?

271 ©2006 AWHONN

Beth (Cont.)

Nurse to Physician/Midwife Reporting

"_____, this is N. Nurse. I am calling to tell you that Beth, a gravida 3 para 1 with an uncomplicated history arrived here about 20 minutes ago. She is in early labor, but we have not been able to detect a fetal heart rate. The resident scanned her and was not able to visualize any cardiac activity."

272 ©2006 AWHONN

Beth (Cont.)

Nurse to Physician/Midwife Reporting (Cont.)

"Beth is having uterine contractions every 2 ½ to 3 ½ minutes, lasting 50 to120 seconds, with coupling. They palpate as mild to moderate. Beth is coping with them and is comfortable. She also is really worried about the status of the baby."

273 ©2006 AWHONN

Beth (Cont.)

Nurse to Physician/Midwife Reporting (Cont.)

"Beth is dilated 4 cm, 80% effaced, -1 station. She had spontaneous rupture of membranes with scant fluid. I need to have you come to the hospital right away."

274 ©2006 AWHONN

Beth (Cont.)

Documentation in Beth's Chart

Toco and US applied. Heart rate tracing shows irregular and bradycardic pattern with uterine contractions. Auscultation with fetoscope. No FHR heard. EFM volume increased, and maternal brachial pulse palpated. HR on monitor synchronous with maternal pulse.

275 ©2006 AWHONN

Beth (Cont.)

Documentation in Beth's Chart (Cont.)

12:15 UC q 2 ½ - 3 ½ min. x 50 -120 sec with coupling. Mild-mod by palpation. Beth very anxious, crying. Husband upset also but trying to comfort her. Charge nurse ___ and ____MD/CNM notified of inability to hear FHR and above findings.

N. Nurse, RN

276 ©2006 AWHONN

Beth (Cont.)

Date of Record: 6/21/2002						
	TIME		12:00			
		:15				
Cervix	Dilation	4				
	Effacement	80				
	Station	-1				
Fetal Heart	Baseline Rate	140s				
	Variability	0				
	Accelerations	0				
	Decelerations	0				
	STIM/pH					
	Monitor Mode					
Uterine Activity	Frequency	q 2.5-3.5				
	Duration	50-120, coupling				
	Intensity	Mild-mod				
	Resting Tone	soft				
	Monitor Mode	Toco/palp				
	Coping	Anxious				
	Maternal Position	lateral				
	O2 L/min/Mask					
	IV					
	Initials					

277 ©2006 AWHONN

Beth (Cont.)

Nurse to Patient Communication

"Beth and Jeff, I just spoke with _____, and
s/he asked me to tell you how concerned s/he
is for you both. S/he wanted me to tell you that
s/he will be here in 10 minutes."

278 ©2006 AWHONN

Remember...

Health care professionals should seek to be familiar
with current guidelines and recommendations
relevant to their practice.

Examples:

- National (laws, regulations)
- State/Provincial (statutes, nurse practice acts)
- Community standards
- Institutional (policies, procedures, protocols)
- Professional associations (practice guidelines)

279 ©2006 AWHONN

Conflict and Conflict Management

- Occasional conflict is a fact of professional life.
- Honest differences of opinion are to be expected.
- At times it may not be possible to resolve these conflicts in a time-frame appropriate to the patient's condition.
- Chain of command is occasionally needed.

280 ©2006 AWHONN

Sample Chain of Command

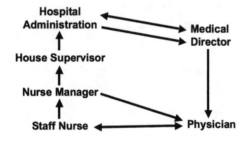

281 ©2006 AWHONN

Evaluation and Synthesis

©2006 AWHONN

Synthesis

- Clear collaborative goals for care
- Physiology and historical data
- Selection/verification of assessment techniques and interventions
- Fetal heart/uterine contraction interpretation
- Timely and effective communication

283 ©2006 AWHONN

The Nursing Process and Fetal Monitoring

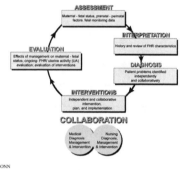

284 ©2006 AWHONN

Pamela, 26 years old
G2 P1001, 39 weeks gestation

- History: Unremarkable
- Current Pregnancy
  - Preeclampsia
  - BP 136/92 - 148/96
  - Sonogram x 2
  - Reactive NST x 3

285 ©2006 AWHONN

Pamela: Admission Assessment

- Admitted for induction of labor for preeclampsia
- Vaginal exam: 3 cm/50%/-2; vertex
- Vital signs: BP 138/88, P 80, R 18, T 98.6 °F (37 °C)
- No contractions, intact membranes

286 ©2006 AWHONN

Pamela: Admission Tracing (0800)

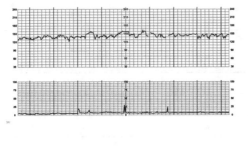

287 ©2006 AWHONN

Does Pamela have any clinically significant risk factors?

288 ©2006 AWHONN

Risks for Decreased Utero-placental Perfusion

- Preeclampsia
- Oxytocin use

289 ©2006 AWHONN

Pamela (Cont.): 1030 (2 1/2 hours later)

290 ©2006 AWHONN

Pamela (Cont.): 1110 (40 minutes later)

291 ©2006 AWHONN

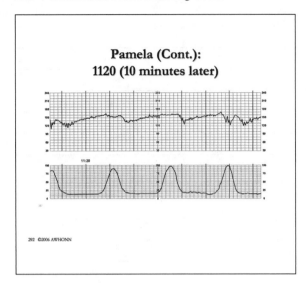

Pamela (Cont.):
1120 (10 minutes later)

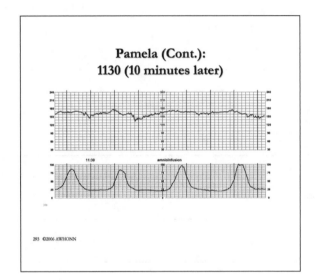

Pamela (Cont.):
1130 (10 minutes later)

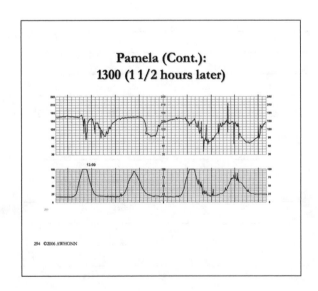

Pamela (Cont.):
1300 (1 1/2 hours later)

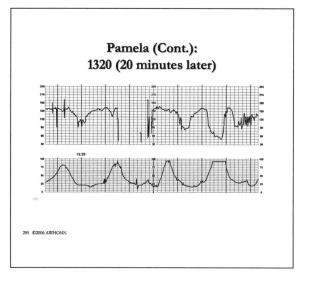

Pamela (Cont.):
1320 (20 minutes later)

295 ©2006 AWHONN

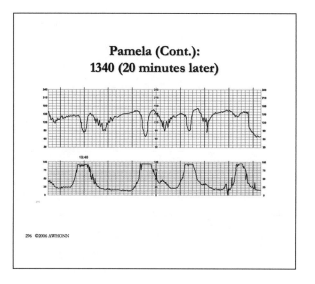

Pamela (Cont.):
1340 (20 minutes later)

296 ©2006 AWHONN

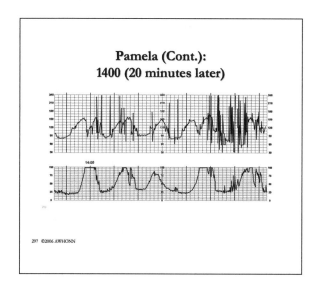

Pamela (Cont.):
1400 (20 minutes later)

297 ©2006 AWHONN

Pamela (Cont.):
1420 (20 minutes later)

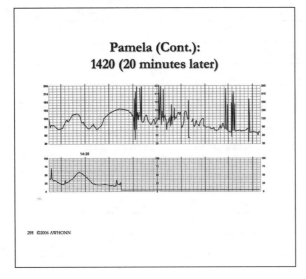

298 ©2006 AWHONN

Pamela - Outcome

Neonatal Outcome

- 5 lbs., 4 oz (2,381 gm) male
- Apgar scores of 3, 7, and 8
  at 1, 5, & 10 minutes
- Arterial cord blood gas values:
  - pH   6.83
  - pCO2   125.0 mmHg
  - pO2   12.4 mmHg
  - BD   22.6 mEq/L

299 ©2006 AWHONN

Key Issues

- Respectful collaboration
- Careful assessment
- Critical decision-making
- Physiologically based interventions
- Evaluation of patterns over time
- Effective communication
- Taking action to resolve difficult situations

300 ©2006 AWHONN

The Nursing Process and Fetal Monitoring

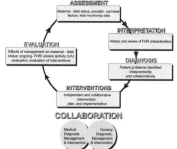

301 ©2006 AWHONN

parasympathetic ↓

sympathetic ↑

STUDENT WORKBOOK

This workbook should be used to document answers for Test B if necessary and the skills stations. Please retain this workbook for your records and do not send it back to AWHONN or Professional Education Services Group.

Intermediate Fetal Monitoring Course Competence Validation

Competence Validation Awarded (participant passed all skill stations and attended the entire workshop)

Instructor's Initials

YES_____ NO_____ Date _____

Skill Stations

Leopold's Maneuvers   PASS_____ FAIL_____ Date _____

Objectives:
1. Explain the purpose of Leopold's maneuvers.
2. Describe patient comfort measures before the procedure.
3. Perform the four steps of Leopold's maneuvers.
4. Identify the optimal site for FHR auscultation on the basis of Leopold's maneuvers.

Auscultation of the FHR   PASS _LFS_ FAIL_____ Date _1/19/09_

Objectives:
1. Choose the appropriate timing of auscultation in relation to uterine contractions.
2. Identify accurate baseline FHR and rhythm.
3. Recognize changes from the baseline as either increases or decreases, as appropriate.
4. Select appropriate interventions to auscultated FHR and rhythm, including when, how and how often you will continue to assess the FHR.

	Cases 1–3	**Cases 4–6**	**Cases 7–9**	**Cases 10–12**
Case Number:	Case # 11	Case # 10	Case # 3	Case # 5
Rate:	160-170	130-140	140's 150-160	130-140's 125-135
Rhythm:	regular	irregular	regular	regular irregular
Interventions:	Apply EFM to obtain more info, reposition,	EFM, reposition notify MD	Continue int. ausc. between and during ctx Q30' good	reposition, apply EFM to obtain more info. good

FSE/IUPC Placement   PASS_____ FAIL_____ Date _____

Objectives:
1. Describe two relative contraindications and two potential risks to placing FSEs and IUPCs.
2. Demonstrate the correct sequence of steps for placing an FSE.
3. Demonstrate the correct sequence of steps for placing an IUPC and ensuring it functions properly.

<u>Communication of Fetal Heart Monitoring Data</u>   PASS _LFS_   FAIL_____   Date _1/19/09_

Objectives: 1. Critique a videotaped scenario of nurse–primary health care provider communication, identifying important points that the nurse in the video omitted.

2. Accurately interpret an EFM tracing and appropriately document the interpretation. Baseline FHR, FHR variability, periodic FHR patterns, episodic FHR patterns and uterine activity must be identified and documented.

3. Document a plan of action or appropriate nursing response that takes into account communication principles, the role and responsibility of the nurse as patient advocate and what to do when a physician or midwife order is not consistent with what you believe to be in the best interest of the woman or her fetus or both.

<u>Integration of Fetal Heart Monitoring Knowledge</u>   PASS _LFS_   FAIL_____   Date _1/19/09_
<u>and Practice</u>

Objectives: 1. Demonstrate appropriate interpretation of the fetal monitor tracing.

2. Demonstrate knowledge of the physiologic mechanisms for the observed patterns.

3. Demonstrate knowledge of instrumentation factors affecting interpretation of the fetal monitor tracing.

4. Demonstrate an understanding of how physiologic mechanisms and interpretation influence the decision-making process.

5. Describe appropriate interventions or management steps for each case scenario.

6. Demonstrate knowledge of evaluation of fetal response to selected interventions.

Exercise I-Documentation Flowsheet

Date of Record: _____					
	TIME				
Cervix	Dilation				
	Effacement				
	Station				
Fetal Heart	Baseline Rate				
	Variability				
	Accelerations				
	Decelerations				
	STIM/pH				
	Monitor Mode				
Uterine Activity	Frequency				
	Duration				
	Intensity				
	Resting Tone				
	Monitor Mode				
	Coping				
	Maternal Position				
	O_2/LPM/Mask				
	IV				
Nurse Initials					

AWHONN FETAL HEART MONITORING PROGRAM

Skill Station: Integration of Fetal Heart Monitoring Knowledge and Practice

Practice Case Answer Sheet

CASE STUDY #____

1. Variability: a. absent (undetectable)   ____

                       b. minimal (>0 but ≤5 bpm)   ✓

                       c. moderate (6–25 bpm)   ____

                       d. marked (>25 bpm)   ____

                       e. unable to determine   ____

2. Baseline FHR: 165

3. Contractions: Frequency   6
                       Duration   110-150
                       Intensity   palpate strong
                       Resting Tonus   palpates relaxed

4. Accelerations and decelerations: When present, circle P if underline{periodic} and E if underline{episodic}.

    Accelerations   P   E
    Early decelerations   (P) E
    Variable decelerations (P) E
    Late decelerations   P   E
    Prolonged decelerations P   E

5. List possible underlying physiologic mechanisms or rationales for observed patterns:

    ~~1. Head compression~~
    2. Cord compression
    Oligo
    old placenta

6. List actions and interventions indicated, based on overall interpretation (physiologic based, instrumentation based and further assessments):

    Position Δ   O2 fluid bolus   support
    amnioinfusion   coping
    call MW and inform   pain + anxiety relief
    compromised MD

© 2006 AWHONN

AWHONN FETAL HEART MONITORING PROGRAM

Skill Station: Integration of Fetal Heart Monitoring Knowledge and Practice

Practice Case Answer Sheet

CASE STUDY #_____

1. Variability: a. absent (undetectable)   _____

     b. minimal (>0 but ≤5 bpm)   _____

     c. moderate (6–25 bpm)   _____

     d. marked (>25 bpm)   _____

     e. unable to determine   _____

2. Baseline FHR: _____

3. Contractions: Frequency   _____

     Duration   _____

     Intensity   _____

     Resting Tonus   _____

4. Accelerations and decelerations: When present, circle P if <u>periodic</u> and E if <u>episodic</u>.

   Accelerations   P   E
   Early decelerations   P   E
   Variable decelerations   P   E
   Late decelerations   P   E
   Prolonged decelerations   P   E

5. List possible underlying physiologic mechanisms or rationales for observed patterns:

6. List actions and interventions indicated, based on overall interpretation (physiologic based, instrumentation based and further assessments):

AWHONN FETAL HEART MONITORING PROGRAM

Skill Station: Integration of Fetal Heart Monitoring Knowledge and Practice

Practice Case Answer Sheet

CASE STUDY #_____

1. Variability: a. absent (undetectable) _____

    b. minimal (>0 but ≤5 bpm) _____

    c. moderate (6–25 bpm) ✓

    d. marked (>25 bpm) _____

    e. unable to determine ✗

2. Baseline FHR: 170

3. Contractions: Frequency _unable to determine_

    Duration _____

    Intensity _____

    Resting Tonus _____

4. Accelerations and decelerations: When present, circle P if periodic and E if episodic.

Accelerations	P	E
Early decelerations	P	E
Variable decelerations	P	(E)
Late decelerations	P	E
Prolonged decelerations	P	(E)

5. List possible underlying physiologic mechanisms or rationales for observed patterns:

    Uteroplacental Insuffiency, cord compression, oligo, old placenta, rapid descent

6. List actions and interventions indicated, based on overall interpretation (physiologic based, instrumentation based and further assessments):

    reposition, vag exam, hydrate, O₂, assess VS call MD

AWHONN FETAL HEART MONITORING PROGRAM

Skill Station: Integration of Fetal Heart Monitoring Knowledge and Practice

Practice Case Answer Sheet

CASE STUDY #_____

1. Variability: a. absent (undetectable)   _____

     b. minimal (>0 but ≤5 bpm)   _____

     c. moderate (6–25 bpm)   _____

     d. marked (>25 bpm)   _____

     e. unable to determine   _____

2. Baseline FHR: _____

3. Contractions: Frequency   _____

     Duration   _____

     Intensity   _____

     Resting Tonus   _____

4. Accelerations and decelerations: When present, circle P if <u>periodic</u> and E if <u>episodic</u>.

     Accelerations   P   E
     Early decelerations   P   E
     Variable decelerations   P   E
     Late decelerations   P   E
     Prolonged decelerations   P   E

5. List possible underlying physiologic mechanisms or rationales for observed patterns:

6. List actions and interventions indicated, based on overall interpretation (physiologic based, instrumentation based and further assessments):

AWHONN FETAL HEART MONITORING PROGRAM

Skill Station: Integration of Fetal Heart Monitoring Knowledge and Practice

Practice Case Answer Sheet

CASE STUDY #____

1. Variability: a. absent (undetectable)   ____

                         b. minimal (>0 but ≤5 bpm)   ____

                         c. moderate (6–25 bpm)   ✓

                         d. marked (>25 bpm)   ____

                         e. unable to determine   ✓

2. Baseline FHR: ~~int~~ 125

3. Contractions: Frequency   1-4
                         Duration   30-90
                         Intensity   palpate
                         Resting Tonus   palpate

4. Accelerations and decelerations: When present, circle P if <u>periodic</u> and E if <u>episodic</u>.

    Accelerations   P   E
    Early decelerations   P   E
    Variable decelerations   (P)   (E)
    Late decelerations   P   E
    Prolonged decelerations   P   E

5. List possible underlying physiologic mechanisms or rationales for observed patterns:

6. List actions and interventions indicated, based on overall interpretation (physiologic based, instrumentation based and further assessments):

© 2006 AWHONN

AWHONN FETAL HEART MONITORING PROGRAM

Skill Station: Integration of Fetal Heart Monitoring Knowledge and Practice

Practice Case Answer Sheet

CASE STUDY #_____

1. Variability: a. absent (undetectable)   _____

                     b. minimal (>0 but ≤5 bpm)   _____

                     c. moderate (6–25 bpm)   _____

                     d. marked (>25 bpm)   _____

                     e. unable to determine   _____

2. Baseline FHR: _____

3. Contractions: Frequency   _____

                     Duration   _____

                     Intensity   _____

                     Resting Tonus   _____

4. Accelerations and decelerations: When present, circle P if <u>periodic</u> and E if <u>episodic</u>.

Accelerations	P	E
Early decelerations	P	E
Variable decelerations	P	E
Late decelerations	P	E
Prolonged decelerations	P	E

5. List possible underlying physiologic mechanisms or rationales for observed patterns:

6. List actions and interventions indicated, based on overall interpretation (physiologic based, instrumentation based and further assessments):

AWHONN FETAL HEART MONITORING PROGRAM

Skill Station: Integration of Fetal Heart Monitoring Knowledge and Practice

Practice Case Answer Sheet

CASE STUDY #_____

1. Variability: a. absent (undetectable)   _____

   b. minimal (>0 but ≤5 bpm)   _____

   c. moderate (6–25 bpm)   _____

   d. marked (>25 bpm)   _____

   e. unable to determine   _____

2. Baseline FHR: _____

3. Contractions: Frequency   _____

   Duration   _____

   Intensity   _____

   Resting Tonus   _____

4. Accelerations and decelerations: When present, circle P if _periodic_ and E if _episodic_.

Accelerations	P	E
Early decelerations	P	E
Variable decelerations	P	E
Late decelerations	P	E
Prolonged decelerations	P	E

5. List possible underlying physiologic mechanisms or rationales for observed patterns:

6. List actions and interventions indicated, based on overall interpretation (physiologic based, instrumentation based and further assessments):

AWHONN FETAL HEART MONITORING PROGRAM

Skill Station: Integration of Fetal Heart Monitoring Knowledge and Practice

Practice Case Answer Sheet

CASE STUDY #_____

1. Variability: a. absent (undetectable)   _____

     b. minimal (>0 but ≤5 bpm)   _____

     c. moderate (6–25 bpm)   _____

     d. marked (>25 bpm)   _____

     e. unable to determine   _____

2. Baseline FHR: _____

3. Contractions: Frequency   _____

     Duration   _____

     Intensity   _____

     Resting Tonus   _____

4. Accelerations and decelerations: When present, circle P if periodic and E if episodic.

Accelerations	P	E
Early decelerations	P	E
Variable decelerations	P	E
Late decelerations	P	E
Prolonged decelerations	P	E

5. List possible underlying physiologic mechanisms or rationales for observed patterns:

6. List actions and interventions indicated, based on overall interpretation (physiologic based, instrumentation based and further assessments):

AWHONN FETAL HEART MONITORING PROGRAM

Skill Station: Integration of Fetal Heart Monitoring Knowledge and Practice

Practice Case Answer Sheet

CASE STUDY #_____

1. Variability: a. absent (undetectable)   _____

b. minimal (>0 but ≤5 bpm)   _____

c. moderate (6–25 bpm)   _____

d. marked (>25 bpm)   _____

e. unable to determine   _____

2. Baseline FHR: _____

3. Contractions: Frequency   _____

Duration   _____

Intensity   _____

Resting Tonus   _____

4. Accelerations and decelerations: When present, circle P if <u>periodic</u> and E if <u>episodic</u>.

Accelerations	P	E
Early decelerations	P	E
Variable decelerations	P	E
Late decelerations	P	E
Prolonged decelerations	P	E

5. List possible underlying physiologic mechanisms or rationales for observed patterns:

6. List actions and interventions indicated, based on overall interpretation (physiologic based, instrumentation based and further assessments):

© 2006 AWHONN

AWHONN FETAL HEART MONITORING PROGRAM

Skill Station: Integration of Fetal Heart Monitoring Knowledge and Practice

Practice Case Answer Sheet

CASE STUDY #_____

1. Variability:
   a. absent (undetectable) _____
   b. minimal (>0 but ≤5 bpm) _____
   c. moderate (6–25 bpm) _____
   d. marked (>25 bpm) _____
   e. unable to determine _____

2. Baseline FHR: _____

3. Contractions:
   Frequency _____
   Duration _____
   Intensity _____
   Resting Tonus _____

4. Accelerations and decelerations: When present, circle P if <u>periodic</u> and E if <u>episodic</u>.

Accelerations	P	E
Early decelerations	P	E
Variable decelerations	P	E
Late decelerations	P	E
Prolonged decelerations	P	E

5. List possible underlying physiologic mechanisms or rationales for observed patterns:

6. List actions and interventions indicated, based on overall interpretation (physiologic based, instrumentation based and further assessments):

AWHONN FETAL HEART MONITORING PROGRAM

Skill Station: Integration of Fetal Heart Monitoring Knowledge and Practice

Practice Case Answer Sheet

CASE STUDY #_____

1. Variability:
    a. absent (undetectable) _____
    b. minimal (>0 but ≤5 bpm) _____
    c. moderate (6–25 bpm) _____
    d. marked (>25 bpm) _____
    e. unable to determine _____

2. Baseline FHR: _____

3. Contractions:
    Frequency   _____
    Duration   _____
    Intensity   _____
    Resting Tonus _____

4. Accelerations and decelerations: When present, circle P if <u>periodic</u> and E if <u>episodic</u>.

Accelerations	P	E
Early decelerations	P	E
Variable decelerations	P	E
Late decelerations	P	E
Prolonged decelerations	P	E

5. List possible underlying physiologic mechanisms or rationales for observed patterns:

6. List actions and interventions indicated, based on overall interpretation (physiologic based, instrumentation based and further assessments):

SKILL STATION
COMMUNICATION OF FETAL HEART MONITORING DATA
PRACTICE PACKET

Please use this page to list your answers for the practice video critique.

Summary	Critique

Nurse to physician reporting omissions

① pt's gest - EDD

② ob hx/complications

③ time of ROM, color fluid

④ dilation? station?
epidural? reason for indx?

PRACTICE

Exercise I

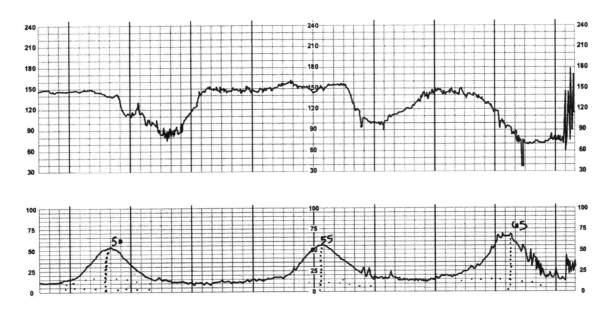

a) Please write a brief description of what you would report to another provider about this tracing:

The pt is having uterine contractractions every 2'½ to 3'½ minutes with an intensity of 50-65 mm/Hg and resting tone of 10-15 mm/Hg. FHR has baseline of 150 with minimal to moderate variability, with late and variable decllerations.

b) Please document your interpretation of this tracing:
- a. Baseline rate   150
- b. Variability   minimal to moderate
- c. Accelerations   none
- d. Decelerations   ~~repetitious~~ late, variable
- e. Uterine activity   Ctx Q 2 - 3'½ min lasting 80-90 sec

Exercise I
Correct Responses

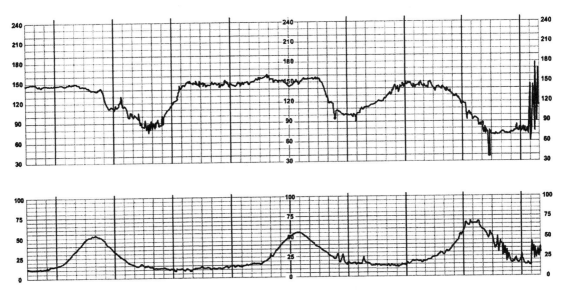

c) Please write a brief description of what you would report to another provider about this tracing:

"The fetal heart rate tracing is showing a mixed pattern of recurrent deep late and variable decelerations. The FHR baseline is currently 150 bpm with moderate variability, but the decelerations are worsening and the patient needs to be seen. Please come to evaluate the patient now. Thank you."

d) Please document your interpretation of this tracing:
   a. Baseline rate _____ 150 bpm _____
   b. Variability _____ moderate _____
   c. Accelerations _____ none _____
   d. Decelerations _____ late and variable _____
   e. Uterine activity _____ q 3–4 min x 60–80 sec_____

Exercise II
Please document your interpretation of the tracing below on the flowsheet provided. The tracing is obtained using a spiral electrode and intrauterine pressure catheter.

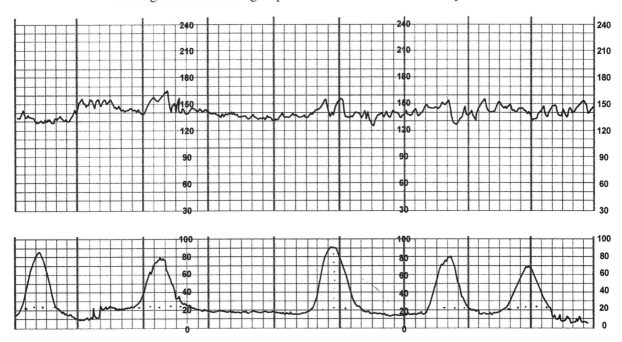

Exercise I-Documentation Flowsheet

Date of Record:	1/20/09				
	TIME				
Cervix	Dilation				
	Effacement				
	Station				
Fetal Heart	Baseline Rate	135			
	Variability	mod.			
	Accelerations	present			
	Decelerations	none			
	STIM/pH				
	Monitor Mode	FSE			
Uterine Activity	Frequency	1 - 2 ½			
	Duration	40 - 50			
	Intensity	40-90 mm/Hg			
	Resting Tone	10-20 mm/Hg			
	Monitor Mode	IUPC			
	Coping				
	Maternal Position				
	O$_2$/LPM/Mask				
	IV				
Nurse Initials					

Exercise II-Correct Documentation

Date of Record: _____					
	TIME				
Cervix	Dilation				
Cervix	Effacement				
Cervix	Station				
Fetal Heart	Variability	Moderate			
Fetal Heart	Baseline Rate	140			
Fetal Heart	Accelerations	Present			
Fetal Heart	Decelerations	Ø			
Fetal Heart	STIM/pH				
Fetal Heart	Monitor Mode	FSE			
Uterine Activity	Frequency	1½–3½ 1			
Uterine Activity	Duration	60–70			
Uterine Activity	Intensity	70–90			
Uterine Activity	Resting Tone	5–20			
Uterine Activity	Monitor Mode	IUPC			
	Coping				
	Maternal Position				
	O_2/LPM/Mask				
	IV				
Nurse Initials					

SKILL STATION:
COMMUNICATION OF FETAL HEART MONITORING DATA TEST

NOTE: There are two separate exercises on this test. Please do both of them.

Exercise I

For this exercise you will watch a video scenario. This scenario can be viewed more than once to answer the question. In viewing the scenario, you will note omissions in the nurse's report. Write down four of the omissions that you hear. There are more than four omissions in the scenario, but you are only required to list four.

good

1. Time of SROM / color of fluid
2. GBS status
3. Current dilation / station / effacement
4. Reason for indx / SROM

Exercise II

Monica is a G3 P2 admitted in early labor at 39 weeks gestation. No risk factors are noted, no antepartum testing was done. She had two previous low-risk pregnancies; these children are now ages 8 and 10. Her vaginal exam reveals a 3 cm, 90% effaced, floating, vertex presentation. Membranes are intact. An US and Toco monitor are in place.

Instructions

A. Interpret the monitor tracings on page 163 and document your findings in two separate columns on the flowsheet provided on page 165.

B. Assume that after the second monitor tracing on page 163 (@1530) you phone in a report to the physician, describing the observed pattern. You are told to call again in one hour if there is no change. Document your short verbal response to the physician in the following space and also describe the next nursing act you will take in response to the physician's order. Take the scenario as far as you believe is appropriate.

Monica's tracing shows absent variability and is non-reassuring. Her ctx pattern is irregular and difficult to trace using the toco. Her ctx palpate mild and are irregular. I will reposition the patient, push an IV fluid bolus and administer O₂ via mask per order to increase uteroplacental bloodflow and fetal umbilical oxygenation, but this tracing is concerning to me and I would like you to come in and assess the patient now. If physician won't come in : "I will follow chain of command"

Exercise II
US, TOCO

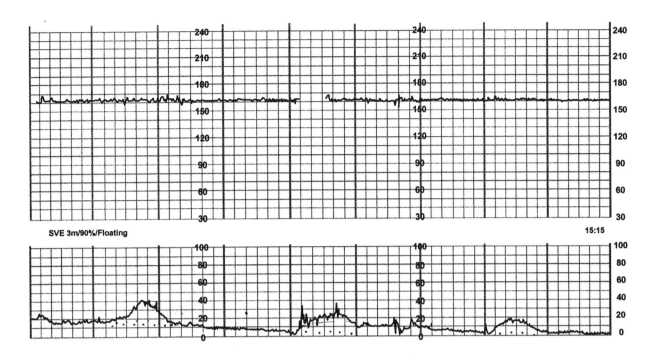

SVE 3m/90%/Floating

15:15

Exercise II, (Continued)
SE, TOCO

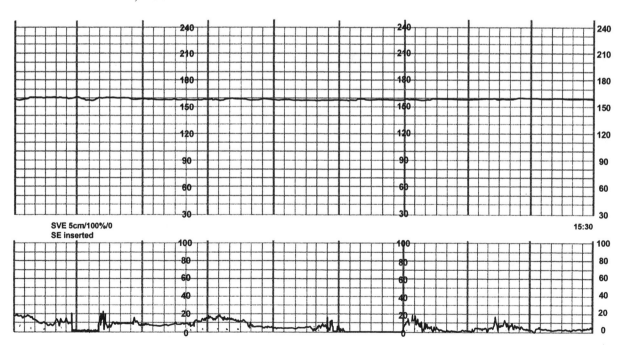

SVE 5cm/100%/0
SE inserted

15:30

Exercise II-Documentation Flowsheet

Date of Record: 1/20/09

	TIME	1507	1515	1522	1530
Cervix	Dilation	3		5	
	Effacement	90		100	
	Station	Floating		Ø	
Fetal Heart	Baseline Rate	160	160	160	160
	Variability	minimal to mod.	minimal	absent	absent
	Accelerations	none	none	none	none
	Decelerations	none	none	none	none
	STIM/pH				
	Monitor Mode	U/S	U/S	FSE	FSE
Uterine Activity	Frequency		3-3½ 3		irregular, 1-2 Toco adjusted
	Duration		60-70 40-60		unable to assess 30-50
	Intensity		mild to palpation		mild to palpation
	Resting Tone		palpates relaxed between ctx		palpates relaxed between ctx
	Monitor Mode	TOCO	TOCO	TOCO	TOCO
	Coping				
	Maternal Position				
	O$_2$/LPM/Mask				
	IV				
	Nurse Initials				

INTERMEDIATE FETAL MONITORING COURSE
TEST B ANSWER SHEET

Participant Name: _____

Test B is to be administered only if the participant does not successfully complete Test A. If the participant successfully completes Test B, Competence Validation will be awarded. If the participants fails both Test A and Test B, Competence Validation should not be awarded.

      Each participant should keep his/her copy of the test booklet and Test B results. The corresponding original questions should be retained by the instructor.

      This form should not be mailed back to the AWHONN processing center.

Answer Sheet

	A	B	C		A	B	C		A	B	C		A	B	C		A	B	C
1	○	○	○	11	○	○	○	21	○	○	○	31	○	○	○	41	○	○	○
2	○	○	○	12	○	○	○	22	○	○	○	32	○	○	○	42	○	○	○
3	○	○	○	13	○	○	○	23	○	○	○	33	○	○	○	43	○	○	○
4	○	○	○	14	○	○	○	24	○	○	○	34	○	○	○	44	○	○	○
5	○	○	○	15	○	○	○	25	○	○	○	35	○	○	○	45	○	○	○
6	○	○	○	16	○	○	○	26	○	○	○	36	○	○	○	46	○	○	○
7	○	○	○	17	○	○	○	27	○	○	○	37	○	○	○	47	○	○	○
8	○	○	○	18	○	○	○	28	○	○	○	38	○	○	○	48	○	○	○
9	○	○	○	19	○	○	○	29	○	○	○	39	○	○	○	49	○	○	○
10	○	○	○	20	○	○	○	30	○	○	○	40	○	○	○	50	○	○	○